# MEN'S HEALTH

First published in June 2020

British Library Cataloguing in Publication Data
A catalogue record for this book is available
from the British Library.

ISBN 978 1 78521 694 7

Library of Congress catalog card no. 2019949573

Published by Haynes Publishing,
Sparkford, Yeovil, Somerset BA22 7JJ, UK
Tel: 01963 440635
Int. tel: +44 1963 440635
Website: www.haynes.com

Haynes North America Inc.
859 Lawrence Drive, Newbury Park,
California 91320, USA

Printed in China

# MEN'S HEALTH

## ALL YOU NEED TO KNOW IN ONE CONCISE MANUAL

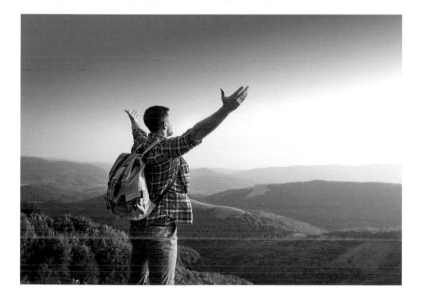

**Jim Pollard**

# Contents

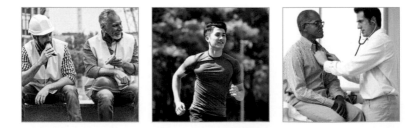

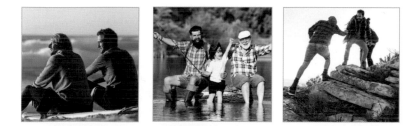

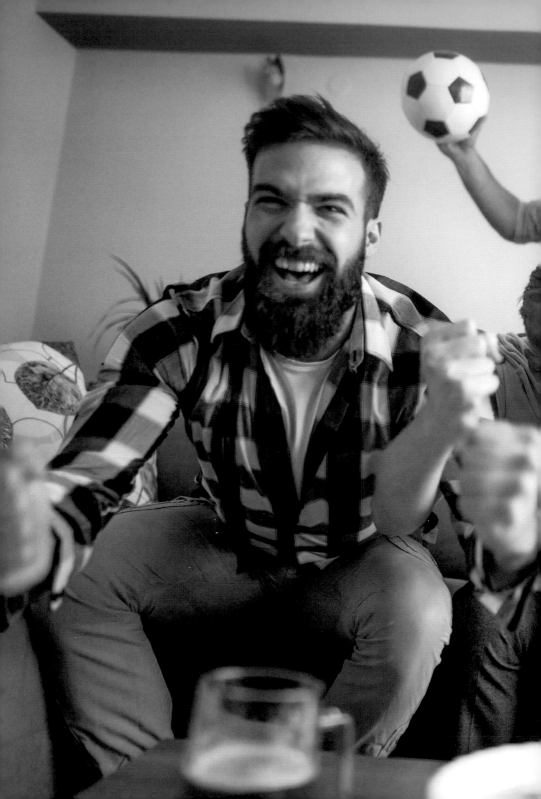

# Who's this book for?

**Can you find your intergluteal cleft?
Or point to your olecranon?**

Of course not. You're like most men when it comes to health, you don't know your arse from your elbow. But don't worry, those are the last medical terms you'll find in this book. From here on, it's plain speaking only.

Since prevention is always better than cure, in this book there are no descriptions of disease, no threats or grim warnings, just a lot of stuff that will help you to be healthier. Easy-going, quick wins for a longer, happier life.

That's some claim for a short book. To be fair, we are living longer anyway. But there's a catch. Although male life expectancy at birth is now close to 80, on average only 63 of those years will be in good health. That's one-fifth of your life in poor health. The aim of this book is to help you to enjoy as many healthy and happy years as possible.

This book is written for all men who are interested in their health and well-being. And all men who are not.

A friend of mine tells this story about a support group he went to after deciding to stop drinking. He wasn't keen. He had a good job, money and a relationship; he didn't feel part of this group of drunks, many of whom had none of these things. But the bloke who took him along encouraged him not to latch onto what was different between him and the other men who spoke but to think about what was the same, to listen out for the words that clicked. It must have worked because he hasn't had a drink since.

I'd take a similar approach to this book. Whatever your age or background, whatever you do or don't do for work, whatever 'sort' of person you think you are, you have something in common with the people in this book. This book is the product of my writing about men's health for over 20 years and talking with men from every walk of life during that time. The insight is theirs.

It's true that generally younger men think less about their health than older ones. Your body lets you wing it when you're young. But that's the physical side. There's evidence that when it comes to mental well-being, younger people are having a tougher time.

That's why this book doesn't just talk about healthy hearts but also about healthy heads. In fact, for me, if you sort out the space between your ears, all the rest follows much more easily. If a physical health problem does come knocking at your door, you'll be far better able to deal with it.

In my case it knocked early. I had cancer at 33. This is very unusual, there are just a few dozen new cases each year in the 30–34 age group. I wasn't expecting it. (I was still winging it.) And I had to learn fast. It would have been handy to have read a book like this beforehand.

Every question in this book has been asked by a man. Read the book straight through or just dip in where you fancy.

**Jim Pollard**

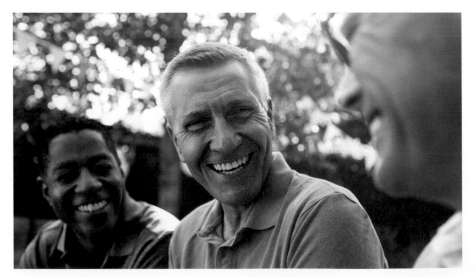

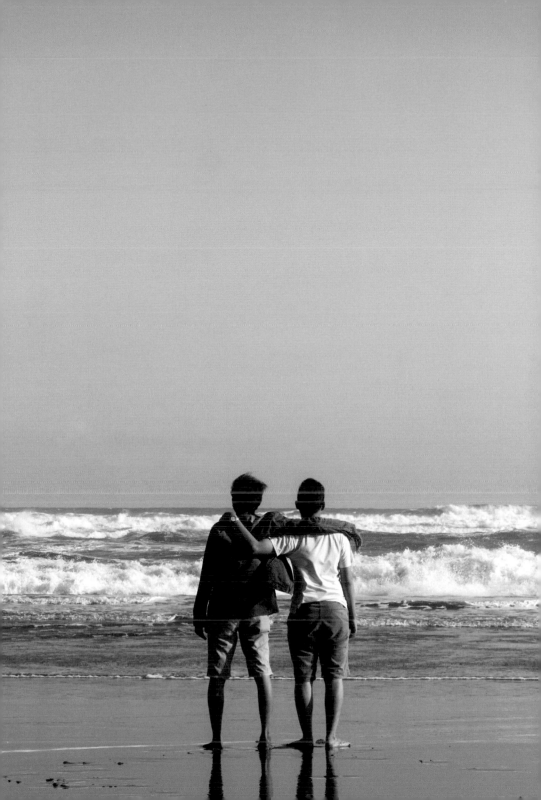

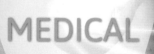

# Chapter 1

# What's the point?

There's no shortage of health advice for men. It starts with your mum and goes from there. This is good for you. That's bad for you. Sometimes both. It's a lot to take in when, for many men, health is not at the top of our priorities. There are other things to do.

Fortunately, like the best technology, the human body is intuitive. It tends to do what you want it to do most of the time, and common sense will get you a long way when it doesn't. However, the human body can easily become old before its time – in the case of the male body, way before its time. One man in five still dies before the age of 65; two in five by the age of 75. It's not necessary.

The male body is not like some sort of computer virus, pre-programmed to self-destruct. But the way we use our bodies and how we fuel them can see them beginning to break down decades sooner than necessary. Unlike your car or laptop, you can't just go out and buy a cheaper, more powerful replacement (although your partner might).

The good news is that compared with even the best tech, the human body is far better designed. Keeping it running smoothly is easy. Anyone can do it. This book explains how, with no medical waffle and no wearable-tech (unless you fancy it).

# So, big changes, right?

No. We're going to see how a few small changes can make a big difference.

## How big a difference?

Good question. Is there any point to all this healthy living stuff? Let's put a number on it. In 2008, the results of a study following 20,000 people over 45 in Norfolk for a decade were published. The researchers gave participants one point for:

- Not currently smoking
- Drinking fewer than 14 units of alcohol per week
- Eating five servings of fruit and vegetables each day
- Not being inactive (that is, taking just half an hour basic exercise a day).

Those who did all four of the above were four times less likely to die during the ten-year study than those who did none of them.

To be more specific, a 60-year-old person with a score of zero had the same risk of dying as a 74-year-old with all four points. So, the answer to the question is that doing all this healthy stuff will add about 14 years to your life. Fourteen years is a lot. That's three World Cups.

Of course, it's not easy to be precise. Everybody is different. But this was no rogue study; research published in 2018 found much the same thing. Adding a fifth healthy behaviour (retaining a healthy body weight), an American study of about 123,000 adults found that those who adopted all five healthy behaviours lived longer: 14 years for women, 12.2 years for men.

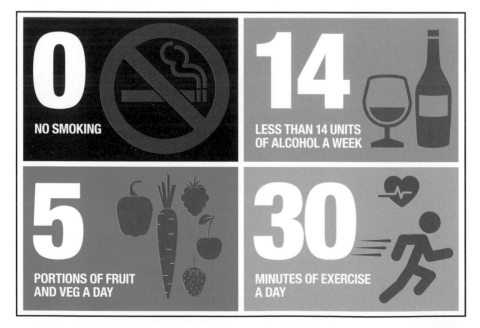

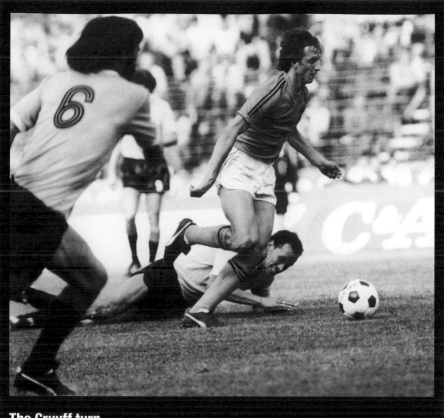

## The Cryuff turn

It's Netherlands v Sweden in the 1974 World Cup. In the 23rd minute, the Dutch captain Johan Cruyff finds himself tightly marked and facing his own goal. He feints a pass but instead scoops the ball back with his instep, pivots 180 degrees on his standing foot and disappears up the pitch leaving both Swedish defender and global audience dumbfounded. The Cruyff turn is born. Kids still learn it today. You don't have to be a football fan to appreciate its balletic beauty.

Why am I talking about Johan Cruyff? It's to help us remember two things. One: he wore the number 14 shirt and 14 is roughly the number of years a healthy lifestyle can add to life expectancy (see page 12) and, two: it's never too late to do your own Cruyff turn.

A heavy smoker, Cruyff had an emergency heart bypass at the age of just 44. He quit the fags. OK, he died of lung cancer in 2016 aged 68 – still way too young – but the Cruyff turn against tobacco effectively bought him another two decades. He once said: 'Football has given me everything in life, tobacco almost took it all away.'

The message: when it comes to healthy changes, the sooner you make them the better, but it's never too late.

## Fourteen years? But isn't health all in the genes?

Genes are a factor, yes, but this research actually proves that simply behaving differently can add years to your life. If you're lucky with your genes too, who knows how long you could go on? Scientists reckon that there's no reason why the human body shouldn't last 120 years or so.

Let's look at the factors that determine our health:

- The hand you're playing (including your genes, age and sex)
- Your lifestyle (which is mostly what this book is about)
- The access you have to services (health, education, etc.)
- Your social and economic position (wealth, work, etc.)
- Your environment (housing, surroundings, etc.).

The first two are by far the most important. True, there's not a lot you can do to change the hand you've been dealt, but you can find out what sort of hand it is by checking your family history. Poker players will tell you that you need to know how good or bad your hand is before even considering whether you want to gamble on it.

Heart disease, cancer and stroke – the biggest killers – run in families. So, often, do mental health problems like depression. Find out whether your parents, grandparents, aunts and uncles have had any of these illnesses, especially if they died young. I had cancer in my thirties. My mum has had cancer and my grandmother died young from it. That simple level of detail is really all you need. Make sure that your GP knows your family health history.

By contrast, your lifestyle is pretty much entirely in your hands. I'm talking about things such as diet, exercise, smoking, drinking, drugs, sexual behaviour, your personality, your attitude to risk, and your attitude to yourself and others. That's what this book is mainly about. To get an idea of the balance between lifestyle and family history, it is estimated that four out of five

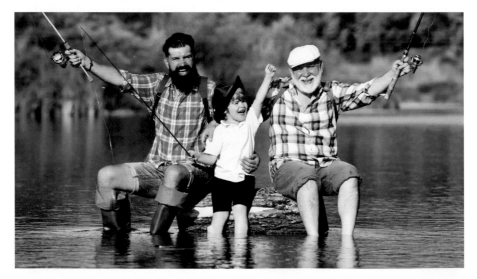

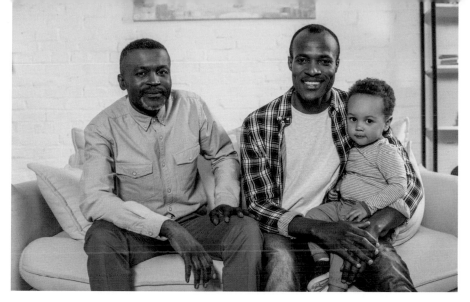

cancers can be prevented. In other words, 80% of cancers are down to lifestyle, so there's a lot you can do.

There's no hard line between lifestyle and genes anyway – lifestyle factors are often the trigger to a genetic predisposition. In other words, lung cancer may be in your genes, but if you don't smoke you may well never trigger it.

## Aren't boys just naturally weaker than girls?

Possibly. Our genetic information – DNA – is carried in our cells in chromosomes. Women have two X chromosomes, which support each other; a flaw in one may be compensated for by the other. Because men have one of each chromosome, an X and a Y, we don't have this built-in support. Hormones may be a factor too. The female hormone, oestrogen, appears to help prevent DNA damage leading to disease. With the male hormone, testosterone, the picture is less positive.

Because levels vary enormously between men and within the same man over the course of the day and over the years, testosterone is hard to study. But it

appears to weaken the immune system and can certainly encourage risky behaviour. Consider this: a study of Korean eunuchs (men castrated as children) found that they lived 14–19 years longer than men with full tackle intact in similar circumstances. Well, it's one way to live longer, I suppose.

Having said all that, we also know that very low levels of testosterone can damage health too – to say nothing of happiness.

So, boys may be a little weaker than girls but the overall impact on life expectancy is minimal. The real impact that being a boy has on your health has little to do with biology and a lot to do with the attitudes and beliefs that many men have.

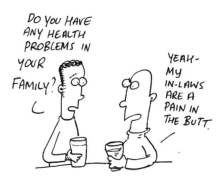

# Attitudes and beliefs

Think back to when you were 8–12 years old. What were the sort of things you heard from adults, other kids, the media, TV and so on about how men are and how they 'should' be? Any of this sound familiar?

- Be strong and silent
- Boys don't cry
- Be self-reliant
- Take risks
- Be courageous
- Be in control
- Be a leader
- Don't ask for help
- Work hard, play hard
- Drink heavily
- Be virile/have a lot of sex.

We could call this the traditional idea of masculinity. These qualities have served the human race well. If you're hunting a wild animal armed only with a spear and a few rocks, if you're descending half a mile into a rickety coal mine with just a flickering headlamp, or if you're about to go over the top to your probable death in the First World War, you need most of these qualities and in large quantities. But the question we need to ask ourselves here is: how many of them are *really* good for your health?

## Isn't it through risk-taking that we make progress?

Definitely. Riding off into the sunset to seek out new worlds and new civilisations is a risk. In fact, many new things, big and small, involve risk. Society can definitely benefit from folk taking risks. It is a part of life and, for whatever reason, men seem to enjoy it. We shouldn't feel bad about this – being male isn't an illness after all – but we do need to understand it.

Perhaps it's hormones, perhaps it's the adrenaline rush, perhaps it's the social

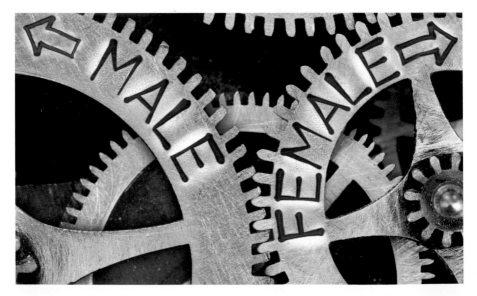

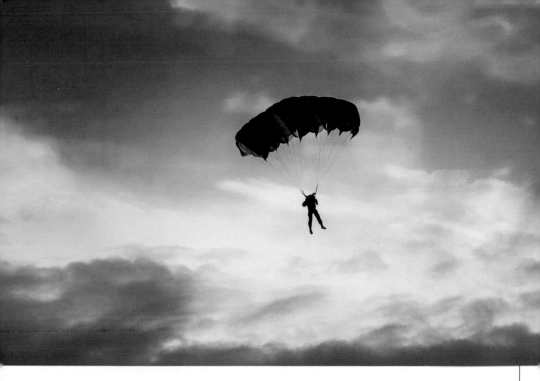

expectations, perhaps it's just fun. There's even some research linking risky behaviour to childhood brain injury.

But, whatever the reason, sometimes these risk-taking impulses combine to make us do some daft and dangerous things. For some men it appears that unless they've actually seen the blood-splattered carnage of a road accident, they can't conceive of just how ugly it might be. This lack of imagination may be very useful before doing battle with a sabre-tooth tiger but it's less helpful when negotiating a supermarket car park.

Risk-taking is normal in adolescence. When you're a teenager you have a sudden rush of hormones pushing you in all directions. At the same time, the parts of the brain that deal with judgement and impulse control haven't yet fully developed. When they do develop, most people grow out of these behaviours. Having said that, you need to be careful about what you get into as a teen. Start to smoke and you'll quickly be a nicotine addict. Start drinking seriously at 14 and your risk of becoming addicted to alcohol is four times greater than if you start at 20. In other words, experimenting as a teenager is fine, but if you adopt a lifestyle at this age it can be difficult to shake off.

We need to get smart. Run risks that are worth running for the right reasons. Find out the facts, make our own choices and be prepared to change our minds when more information comes along. These are far more useful skills, ones that will be valued more highly by men and women alike. Nobody is saying that you shouldn't jump out of a plane – just think about it for long enough to make sure that you've got your parachute on and know how to use it. When it comes to the risks you run with your health, this book is that parachute!

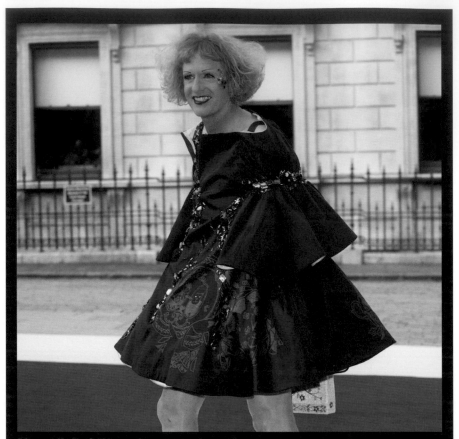

## Masculinity? It's a skeuomorph, mate

The artist Grayson Perry, known for his gender-busting costumes, has an interesting take on all this masculinity business.

The designs of stone buildings often use features that look like supports and struts: a visual reminder of the wooden buildings that came before them. This sort of salute to the past is called a skeuomorph. You can also see skeuomorphs on your favourite tech: the retro envelope on your email app is a reminder of the physical communication – sending letters – that email has replaced.

Grayson Perry sees traditional masculinity in the same way: it may have served a purpose once upon a time but it no longer has much use. We're clinging on to a skeuomorph. You only have to compare the attitudes across the generations to see how ideas of what it is to be a man are changing. And it's never too late for us, as individuals, to change our attitudes. We can be proud of what our fathers and grandfathers did, but we don't have to be like them. In fact, we owe it to the next generation to not be like them.

## So, is masculinity 'toxic' or in 'crisis'?

I'm not sure how useful all this kind of jargon is. Not a lot, probably. But to me, masculinity may risk becoming toxic – by which I mean dangerous to society – when it emphasises some of the qualities or stereotypes of traditional masculinity to the exclusion of others.

One thing all those roles I mentioned earlier – hunter, miner, soldier – had in common is that they were about working with others for a greater good: meat for the tribe, fuel for industry, peace in Europe. Take the wider good out of masculinity and it can become selfish, narrow and even racist or misogynistic.

The fact is, most of the differences we see between men and women are social and cultural rather than biological. Don't let ideas of what a man should be imprison you or those around you. Be who you want to be. Be yourself.

## What's this really got to do with health?

Research shows that men who have these very traditional attitudes and behaviours have poorer health outcomes than men who don't. The danger in believing that it is not manly to ask for help is obvious enough when it comes to health care. But these traditional ideas can also lead to heavy drinking, recklessness and aggression, leading in turn to accidents, violence and a lack of self-care. Even food can become gendered, with men tending to see red meat – perhaps the least healthy protein option – as more masculine.

Change your attitudes, change your behaviour, change your health outcomes.

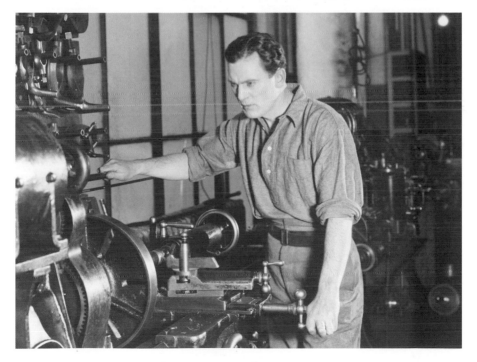

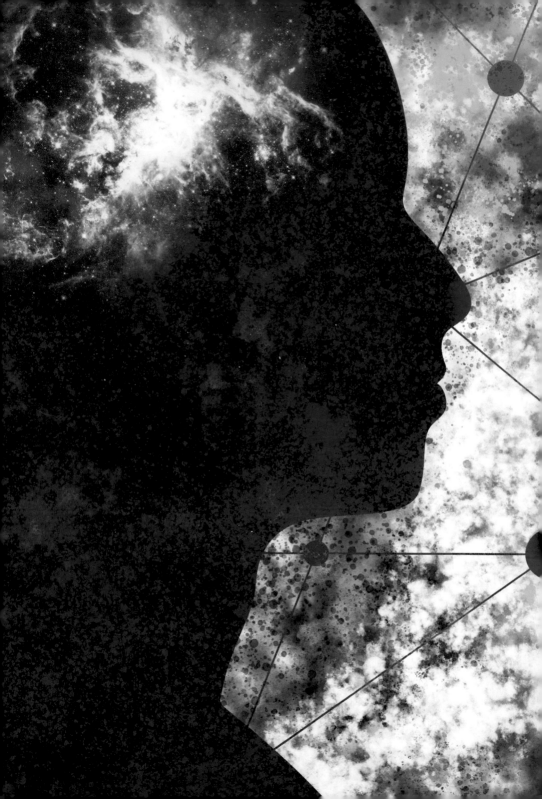

# Chapter 2

# Head first

If you only read one chapter of this book, read this one. It's called 'Head first' for the simple reason that the most important part of the body when it comes to good health is not your heart or your lungs but your head. The muscle that really counts is between your ears.

Don't worry, all the stuff about diet and exercise and improving your sex life is coming up, but just bear with me for a bit.

Good health isn't about jogging every day, or eating tons of vegetables, or even about giving up smoking – although all of these things will help. It's about feeling comfortable in your own skin. Being content within yourself will considerably reduce your chances of having heart attacks, cancer or other major health problems.

What's more, if you are affected by a health problem (and you will be, eventually), this sense of well-being within yourself will help you to cope with it a lot better than you would have otherwise. In the meantime, you'll get a lot more out of life.

# The five ways to well-being

There's lot of research, but it drills down to this: there are five ways to well-being. Developed as part of a serious slab of research by the New Economics Foundation, the five ways to well-being are simple evidence-based ideas that any of us can tap into. Exactly the sort of quick, easy wins I'm talking about. In the short term, they will make us feel better; in the long term, they will help us deal more readily with any mental health challenges we might face. In other words, the five ways are for anyone at any time – not just when you're feeling down or worse. These are the five ways.

### 1  CONNECT

Make contact with others and keep it as frequent and 'real' as possible. Try:

- Talking to someone, rather than texting or emailing
- Talking to someone new – a neighbour or workmate, perhaps
- Asking someone something you've never asked them before
- Offering someone a lift or suggesting you travel together
- Calling someone you haven't spoken to for over a year.

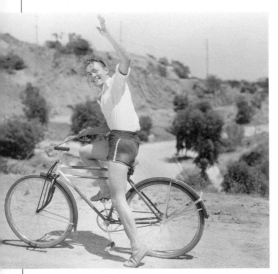

### 2  (BE) ACTIVE

Regular physical activity eases depression and anxiety. Every little helps. There's a full section on this on page 41.

### 3  (TAKE) NOTICE

Yep, it just means noticing what's around you, enjoying your environment. Try:

- Looking up: skies and rooftops not pavements
- Getting a plant or three
- Tidying your desk
- Taking a different route on a familiar journey
- Going somewhere new for lunch
- Getting out into the green (park, common, countryside, etc.) or by water (lake, seaside, etc.). As well as your daily dose of vitamin D (which a lot of us don't have enough of), it also helps boost mood and energy levels. Take a particular interest in something you find there – plants, trees, birds, butterflies, berries. How many different types do you see? It's amazing how much is out there if we are just open to seeing it.

### 4  LEARN (OR DISCOVER)

Keep learning, whatever your age. It's good for self-esteem and social interaction.

But it's also good exercise for the brain and can help boost memory and cognitive skills. Try:

- Signing up for a class
- Reading a book
- Doing some puzzles
- Researching something you're curious about (family tree, perhaps?)
- Taking up a language or a musical instrument
- Learning some practical skills such as cooking or fixing your bike
- Being original – what about a small new thing every day? A new route to work, a new cafe, a new fruit, a different newspaper, a new website, a new app, new music….

## 5  GIVE (OR OFFER)

We all know that giving helps us feel better about ourselves. Why do we sometimes find it so difficult to do? Try:

- Volunteering – a change is as good as a rest so if you sit down for work, perhaps choose something more physical
- Visiting an elderly neighbour or relative
- Giving some of your old 'junk' to charity
- Joining a community group – being part of a group is known to boost well-being. It can be anything from art to Zumba, but make it local (bonus points: become one of the organisers)
- Doing someone a favour
- Thanking someone
- Smiling

The idea that just saying 'thanks' can make us feel better sounds daft but there's good evidence for it. The catch is: you have to mean it. You could put it in writing. Every day note down one thing you're

grateful for, big or small. Or write it on a piece of paper and put it in a jar. Writing it down will make you feel better. Later, if you feel down, read them.

If you want an easy way to remember the five ways, my colleague Tez Cook came up with this: CAN DO. See what he did there? C(onnect), A(ctive), N(otice), D(iscover) and O(ffer). Works for me. A variation is GLANCE with the E standing for etc. – a reminder that the five ways are only a starting point and you can add more.

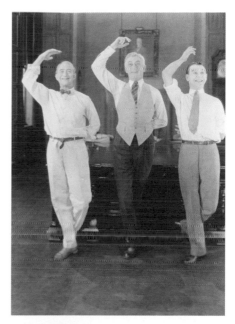

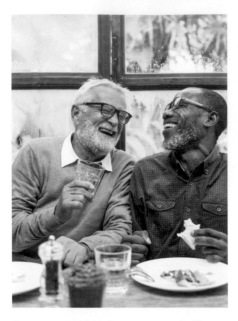

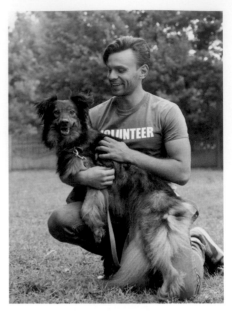

## Are you saying happy people live longer? My Great Uncle Alan is the grumpiest sod you'll ever meet and he's 93

Happiness is good for you because if you're happy you're more likely to do the things that are good for you like eat well, sleep well and exercise. Research also suggests that happiness can boost the immune system, help fight infections and reduce the levels of the hormone cortisol produced when we are stressed. High cortisol levels can lead to disturbed sleep, weight gain, high blood pressure and diabetes. This means happiness may help protect the heart and increase life expectancy. How much these benefits are down to just feeling happy and how much to the healthy behaviours that result is less clear, but either way happiness is healthy.

One study found that unhappy people were 14% more likely to die than very happy people – that magic number 14 again. A specific thing that might help

Great Uncle Alan is laughter. There's evidence that it's good for heart and mood, releasing all sorts of positive hormones like dopamine and serotonin.

One study even suggested 20 seconds of good hard belly laughter was worth three minutes on the rowing machine. Your favourite sit-com, a dodgy joke on WhatsApp… laughing with others (not at them) works best because hearing others laugh triggers feel-good feelings in us. The great thing about the health-boosting power of laughter is that it doesn't have to be genuine. Fake laughter works too. Even a fake smile can lower your heart rate and make you feel better.

### Quick Win

#### Animal Magnetism
*Looking after pets, stroking or patting them, boosts mental wellbeing and lowers blood pressure. Even looking at fish in an aquarium helps you relax.*

# MARK: MY WAYS TO WELL-BEING

When I went to the optician I was expecting a new pair of glasses. It wasn't like that at all.

Apparently, the pressure in my eyes was off the charts. The optician said, 'You need to go to hospital right now.' I was told I needed immediate treatment and would lose the sight in my left eye. It was a real shock. I was 40 years old.

We had three kids at home and one on the way. Work were brilliant at first but my sight was getting worse. They let me go. I wasn't too down as the DWP said there was lots they could do for me. That turned out not to be so. I began to think I wouldn't work again: a big knock-back.

We had a lot on credit cards and needed debt counselling to get it consolidated. It was humiliating. I started drinking more. It was OK at first, a couple of nights a week. Then it creeps up. Every night. Then during the day too. I started withdrawing. I'd lock myself in the bedroom with a few beers and my music. This went on for three years, I suppose. I was verbally nasty to my partner, putting her down to make me feel better. But it didn't make me feel better, I felt worse. I was close to losing her. I knew I was.

We had a massive row. I said: 'I've got to stop drinking.' I went back to my mum's and stayed there for a fortnight. My partner wasn't sure she could trust me, but I knew I wouldn't drink. Something clicked. I just wanted to be with her and the kids. The GP put me in touch with Addaction.

I thought stopping drinking would make all the difference, but Addaction helped me realise I was drinking for a reason. I was feeling guilty, angry and I was depressed. They offered one-to-one counselling and then group sessions. They took me to the gym. An instructor introduced me to another member who was blind. He had no sight at all but had been coming for years. He encouraged me. I joined a couple of classes to get to know people. Now I go five times a week, usually with a mate. We have a good chat.

I was still bored sometimes and a friend suggested voluntary work. A charity shop was out. My partner said I was a good listener and suggested Samaritans. They were positive from the outset. They didn't have any blind volunteers but said 'we'll find a way'. That put a bounce in my step.

I often felt that I was a burden on others but that feeling left once I started volunteering. I do a couple of shifts a week and I'm a group leader. I feel productive. Valued. Like I'm giving something back to my community. It makes my brain function. And it puts things in perspective. I am really lucky with my family and friends.

Both Addaction and Samaritans helped me understand how important talking and listening is. I'm more honest now about how I feel. I still have my moments, but I tell my partner about my frustrations. I don't look back with rose-tinted spectacles.

# Hard talk

Talking often lets us see the solution for ourselves in a way that thinking alone can't. Of course, thinking about stuff is important, but talking about it pushes us into being more truthful. Once something is said, it's out there. You can see what it really is. It's not just a swirling mass of thoughts in your head. (Writing it down helps in a similar way.)

## Why is talking so difficult?

Partly it's about all those attitudes and beliefs about what it means to be a man. We've all heard them, men and women, so it's not surprising we're a bit reluctant to open up. When it comes to health, there's a more practical reason too. Generally, men are pretty lucky with their bodies. Big changes at puberty but then, for most of us, nothing much – not for a while, anyway. Women also have big changes at puberty but then every month, changes in their bodies affect how they feel physically and emotionally. All we have to do is shave.

The downside of this is that we are not used to talking about our bodies or our feelings because a lot of the time we don't have to. When something does happen, we don't know what to say. We don't

mention it. Hope it will go away. Today, parents and teachers are encouraged to discuss feelings with children, to give them the words and the confidence to talk about them. It's an important lesson for all of us.

## We've got by for years without talking about feelings

Times change and we're fools if we don't notice. The brain is not only the most important muscle when it comes to health, it is also the most important muscle when it comes to work. In the UK today, far more jobs require hard thinking than heavy lifting. Reason enough to take what's going on between your ears more seriously.

But being aware of your own feelings is about more than getting a better job. When things happen, we feel them. And,

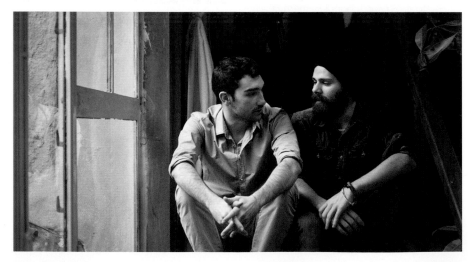

whether or not we choose to take notice of those feelings, they will still affect us.

Senior police officer John Sutherland puts it really well. John had severe depression and a breakdown (you can read about it in his excellent book, *Blue*). He talks about what is known in police forensics as Locard's exchange principle, the idea that every contact leaves a trace. Dr Locard was referring to contact between criminal and victim, but looking back on the build-up to his breakdown, John applies the idea to life in general. Things that happen to you will affect you: every contact leaves a trace. Perhaps more so when you're younger. But also throughout your adult life. We might like to pretend it's all water off a duck's back. But the truth is that experiences, good and bad, leave a trace. They affect us. You can choose to ignore feelings but you can't choose not to have them.

Perhaps men in the past could get away with it. But in today's fast-moving world where we all seem to be 'on' all the time, the contacts (and their traces) come thick and fast.

Rudyard Kipling's popular poem 'If' – the one that ends with the line 'you'll be a man, my son' – urges men to 'meet with Triumph and Disaster and treat those two impostors just the same.' You might want to treat them the same but that doesn't mean that they are the same. Or that you should not notice the differences between them. We need to think about the things that happen to us: good, bad and ugly; be honest with ourselves about how we feel about them; and, yes, talk about them.

John Sutherland's experience is more evidence that nobody, no matter how tough they or their job may be, is immune from mental health challenges. Because John

## Anger management

Anger is normal and inevitable. Doing some of the things in this book might reduce its frequency and intensity – that's good – but sooner or later, the red mist will fall. Three things that can help when it does:

1 **Take control** – The most power you ever have is in the moment between when someone says or does something to you and when you react to it. At this point you can choose any response you like. Use that time. Think before you react.
2 **Walk away** – Walking away is a very easy win. Next time you're in an argument, try it. It won't just help your blood pressure but your sense of being in control too.
3 **Three minute time out** – A simple mindfulness exercise you can use when stressed or angry can really help. If you don't know one, search: '3 minute breathing space'.

wasn't examining his feelings too much, his depression crept up on him as stealthily as a thief and he didn't really notice it until he was in A&E. When it comes to feelings, we need, as the coppers on the beat used to say, to keep 'em peeled.

Watch out for the warning lights on the dashboard (see page 133). The sooner we're aware of a mental health problem, the easier it is to deal with. Everyone's experience is different, of course, but the one thing we can say for certain is that if you ignore mental health warning signs they will only get worse. Eventually, you will break down.

# Stress test

We tend to use the word 'stress' to describe everyday pressures. But in science, stress testing involves pushing something like a building material or computer software to its limits to see when it cracks. Worth bearing in mind here.

For the human being, a little stress is normal, even useful. It may help focus the mind to have the pressure of a deadline, for example. But too much is unhealthy.

## How do I know what's too much?

We're all different. But the more aware you are of your feelings, the easier this question will be to answer for you.

The Holmes–Rahe scale may help. It was developed in the 1960s by psychiatrists Thomas Holmes and Richard Rahe. It won't help you predict illness but it does give a good idea of the impact the stress caused by different life events can have on your physical and mental health.

The scale gives points for different events. The more points you acquire, the higher your risk of subsequent illness. Holmes and Rahe's findings suggested

that if you scored over 150 in any one year, you were at a 50% higher risk of a stress-related illness: further evidence that every experience leaves its mark, whether we choose to notice it or not.

You might wonder how they can give such precise numbers with any accuracy and I'd agree. (Is separating from your partner really worse than jail?) But the point is, it gets us thinking about the stress in our lives. These major episodes are not the only causes. The background hum of stress takes its toll. Further down the Holmes–Rahe list are things you may hardly notice. They include things at work like: a change in work habits (20), trouble with an employer (23), more or less responsibility at work (29) and a change in line of work (35). All of these are on the increase in today's insecure job market. And they all add up.

## The Holmes–Rahe scale: top 10

| | | |
|---|---|---|
| 1 | Death of partner (or child) | 100 |
| 2 | Divorce | 73 |
| 3 | Marital separation | 65 |
| 4 | Going to jail | 63 |
| 5 | Death of close relative | 63 |
| 6 | Serious illness or injury | 53 |
| 7 | Marriage | 50 |
| 8 | Losing job | 47 |
| 9 | Marital reconciliation | 45 |
| 10 | Retirement | 45 |

**Quick Win**

*Take a break*
*Take a screen break if you're working at a computer: a five-minute break every hour and longer breaks every three hours or so. Good for health, breaks will also improve decision-making, productivity and creativity. It's even better if you actually move. Get up from your desk, walk, stretch a little. Take your lunch break (and perhaps use it to go for a walk).*

We sometimes hear someone claim that stress doesn't bother them at all. This is simply not true, unless they have had a part of their brain removed. You may not react outwardly or immediately, but feel it you will. The individuals who handle stress best are not those who kid themselves that they don't let it in, but those who know how to let it out again.

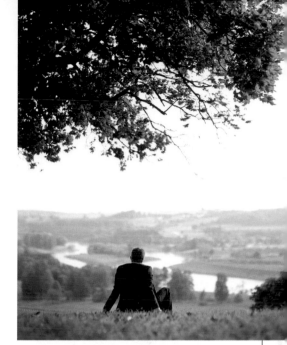

## So have you got any stress reduction techniques?

Here are ten, all backed by evidence. The five ways to well-being on pages 22–23 will help you come up with more.

1 **Try a change of scenery** – Get out to where the air is sweeter and the landscape greener.

2 **Have a swim** – Any physical exercise will do but, when you add the relaxing effect that just looking at water can have, swimming is a top stress buster.

3 **Be childlike** – Rediscover the kid inside you and enjoy games, play and silly jokes.

4 **Laugh** – See page 24.

5 **Read** – Dive into a book (this book, for example), a better stress-busting escape than TV. Reading in the evening also helps relaxation and sleep.

6 **Dance** – Again, any physical activity helps reduce stress by triggering neurotransmitters and endorphins, but dancing is fun (especially if done with someone else) and (if you're doing proper steps) it also occupies the mind.

7 **Sing** – The breathing control required in singing is a natural stress-buster that will get you breathing normally and thinking clearly again.

8 **Have sex** – Making love gets the heart and the hormones going, helps you to sleep and reduces irritability. (If your stress is caused by time pressures, it's perfect because, according to the famous Kinsey report, 75% of men finish within two minutes.)

9 **Have (or give) a massage**

10 **Do nothing** – For five minutes a day, sit or lie down, put some music on if you like, but don't actually do anything. Relax. Not as easy as it sounds but worth it. If you like it, check out mindfulness and meditation.

### Quick Win

**Be a kid**
*Think of something, a creative activity perhaps, that you used to enjoy as a child but don't do any more and do it. Painting, drawing, Lego, a computer game, skipping. It will feel silly at first. Give yourself at least half an hour.*

# Nudge yourself

In the 1990s, the designers of Schiphol Airport in Amsterdam made a revolutionary addition to the gents' toilets that supposedly reduced urine spillage by 80%. No, it wasn't a big sign saying 'don't pee on the floor'. They printed an actual-size image of a housefly on the inside of the urinals. Men had something to aim at and voila... pee-free floors.

A whole industry has grown up out of this sort of idea. It's sometimes called nudge theory: steering people in a direction they probably want to go in anyway while maintaining their freedom of choice.

Traditional public health messages have been a bit like someone in a white coat shouting at you from the sidelines. 'Do this!' 'Don't do that!' Nobody really likes being shouted at, so something more subtle has obvious appeal. The NHS has tried it. When texts reminding patients of

their next appointment also informed them of the cost of a missed appointment, it reduced no-shows by 3% – a statistically small but financially significant improvement when you remember how many people the NHS treats.

There are other examples of health nudges. Ingenious designers have come up with all sorts of ways to encourage people to use the stairs, such as making them look like a piano keyboard or a running track or even printing every couple

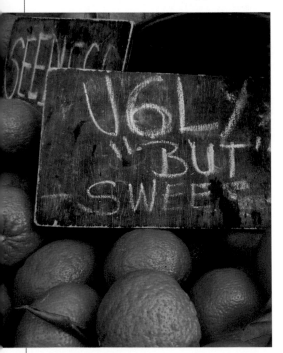

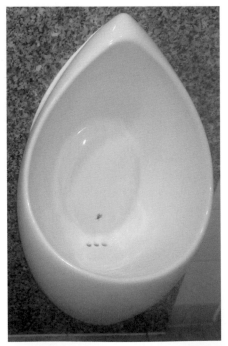

of steps: one calorie burned, two calories burned and so on. Changing how food is displayed, using arrows to point shoppers to the vegetables and offering take-away customers the chance to downsize a meal (rather than upsize it) have all been tried with some success.

Researchers reckon that adding information to food labels about what you need to do to burn off the calories in the food can nudge us into healthier choices. A fizzy drink containing 138 calories, for example, could be accompanied by a symbol showing it takes 26 minutes to walk off. In a study, participants selected 65 fewer calories per meal when these so-called exercise-based labels were included.

A good health nudge should make the desired choice easier or less effort and/or motivate you to make that choice. So, can we nudge ourselves?

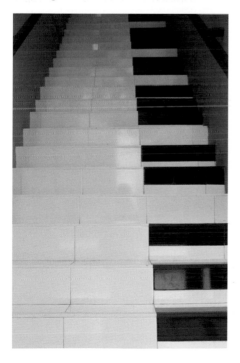

Many smokers, including me, have used a basic nudge to help us quit. You simply put to one side each day the money you would have otherwise spent on fags and watch the pile grow. What will you spend it on?

So, thinking about a health change that you want to make, what sort of nudge might help? A financial incentive or something a bit more subtle? Obviously the better you understand yourself, the better you can nudge yourself. Here are ten ideas:

1  **Hide the biscuits** – Put the biscuit tin in a really awkward place and have a bowl of fruit by the telly instead.
2  **Use smaller plates** – In one experiment, when plate sizes in hotel restaurants were reduced by 2 inches, food waste was reduced by 22%. Guest satisfaction remained the same. Do it at home and as well as reducing your waste, you'll reduce your waist.
3  **Don't keep your favourite tipple at home** – You're not banning yourself from drinking beer or wine or whatever (banning something may actually make us crave it more), you're just ensuring

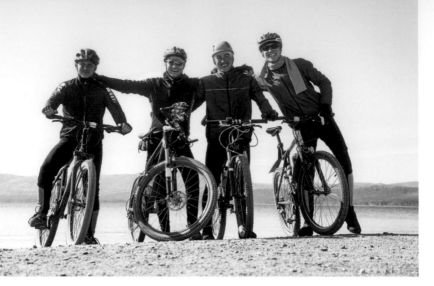

that you have to leave the house to enjoy it. Ice cream or cake might be other candidates for the not-at-home treatment.

4   **Buy cheap kit** – If you never go out on your beloved bicycle because you're worried that someone will nick it, buy a cheap bike and use that around town.

5   **Reduce the amount of preparation you need** – Going for a walk wearing what you're standing up in is easier than getting all your running gear on or finding your swimming costume.

6   **And, if you do need kit for your chosen activity, keep it accessible** – Cupboard by the door, maybe. At work. Perhaps have more than one set of kit. Boot of the car works for some (but again, don't buy a load of expensive stuff you daren't leave there).

7   **Get an app you like** – Even a simple pedometer that counts your steps may be all the encouragement you need to walk a little further.

8   **Find some competition** – If you find that competing against yourself by timing yourself or counting motivates

you, do it. If you want to compete against others, there are clubs and umpteen online options: apps, websites, online programmes.

9   **Pay in advance** – Not wanting to waste your money may motivate you. For me, it means I see my yoga class as a fixed event in my diary, not just something I may turn up to if I'm around and fancy it. True, this often doesn't seem to work for gym memberships: many expire virtually unused. But a specific class at a specific time with specific people that you've already paid for might.

10  **Exercise with others** – The wish not to let others down might motivate you, if you're the fourth for tennis or badminton doubles, for example.

## Quick Win

### *Choose your friends*
*There is evidence that we're more likely to smoke or put on weight if our friends do. This applies to positive changes too. Find new friends or team up with your existing mates to change together.*

# Crisis? What crisis?

### Am I having a mid-life crisis?

OK, let's not talk about crisis, let's talk about change. What we're talking about here is a move from one phase of your life to another. Shakespeare talks about the seven ages of man in *As You Like It*. Crisis implies something bad. But this change needn't be. In the long term, this 'crisis' may be the best thing that's ever happened to you.

The word crisis also suggests something unexpected. But this is nearly as predictable as puberty. Both may be difficult but neither are unusual. You could argue that the 'mid-life crisis' is best seen as the psychological version of wisdom teeth – the last bit of growing up. But mid-life is not strictly accurate either. Some people talk about a quarter-life crisis now. Truth is we probably have a number of

periods when we are moving from one phase of our life to another.

The thing is that when we're young we're seldom as smart as we think we are and we certainly don't know ourselves very well. Yet we make some big decisions. Many of us make choices that don't reflect who we really are and what we value. We do things our parents want, we follow careers we think are respectable or lucrative rather than because we want to, we mistake love for lust, and form partnerships on the basis of a hormonal roller coaster which – although wonderful – can only ever be short term.

That's how adult life begins for us all and, within the space of a few short years, we suddenly find ourselves playing all these adult roles while still feeling like kids inside. Perhaps, we tell ourselves, we'll grow into it. Maybe. Or maybe something's got to give.

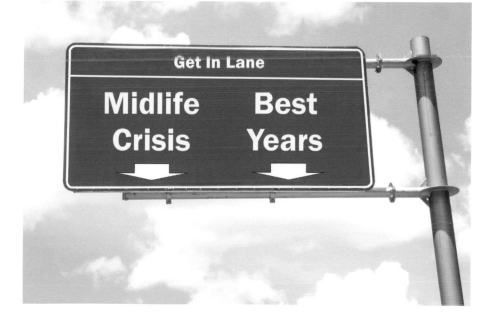

## So the crisis is not the invention of modern society?

No, it is not, although it sometimes looks like it. Life used to be nasty, brutish and short, but now we have these things called choices.

You could see what we're talking about here as an internal conflict between the choices you made and the choices you

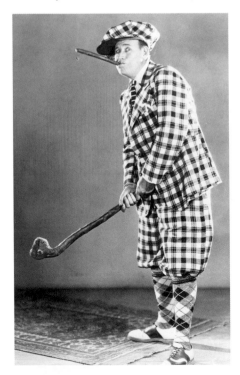

wish you'd made (or would have made had you known yourself better), the conflict between the life that you're living, the roles that you're playing and what you truly are.

## Doesn't sound like 'the best thing ever'...

The next phase of your life could be great if it's based on knowing yourself better, knowing what makes you happy, making choices based on your values and desires and not anyone else's. It is not easy or always affordable, but it's possible. This is why some of today's retired generation are having the time of their lives.

There's no right or wrong about this. People can experience this 'crisis' at any time and some people more than once. For some it might be painful to them and to those around them. Others move more gently from one phase of their life to another. Some lucky souls whose first adult choices were pretty similar to their true natures may never be troubled by any of this at all.

The reason the crisis occurs in mid-life for lots of people is that many of the triggers that can force us to start looking seriously at ourselves and our lives also happen in mid-life. Careers and relationships can stagnate and not live up to our expectations. Geographical mobility can leave us further from our roots. Children become more independent. Parents get old. If that's not enough, the aches and pains in our own body serve as a daily reminder of our own mortality. Perhaps more than any other trigger, it is the grudging acceptance of the inevitability of our own appointment with death that gives us the kick up the arse we need – it's now or never.

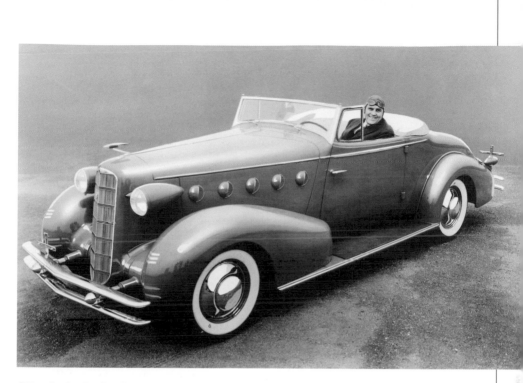

### OK – but why buy a sports car?

Initially, the things that must be done 'now or never' may appear pretty pathetic to a non-male: buying a sports car, taking up an extreme sport or having an affair, for example. What is going on is that we're trying to revisit the choices we made when we were younger.

However, if those revisited choices are still based on poor self-knowledge, mistaken premises and inherited assumptions, then they won't be any better than the first time and probably worse. A man who has learned nothing may well find himself repeating the mistake of choosing a long-term partner on the basis of immediate sex appeal.

Our aches and pains and all they herald for the future are not the only physical trigger of the crisis. For men, the hormone that once got us chasing after all those goals with such enthusiasm is on the wane.

Testosterone levels begin to fall from around the age of 40. Testosterone replacement therapy (TRT) may help for a while but it's only delaying the inevitable. Of course, declining testosterone is scary, especially for men who have always done most of their thinking with their libidos. The art is to see this 'crisis' as a great opportunity to think about something else instead. (See page 105 for more on TRT.)

(See page 105 for more on TRT.)

> **Quick Win**
>
> ### Stop buying new
> *Nobody wants to waste the planet's resources. Reusing and recycling feels good. Online or through charity shops, you can give, get or buy cheaply everything from clothes to furniture. Feeling good and saving money – no wonder there are so many TV programmes on this theme.*

# Mind games

## How can I improve my memory?

Use it. That means actively trying to remember things you want to remember rather than just hoping that you do. Here are five ways to develop a better memory:

1 **Use more than one sense** – Reproducing information helps it stick:

   ■ If someone tells you something, write it down. The evidence is that you'll remember and understand better if you make written notes. You might record more if you type, but by writing it, your brain begins processing the information right away.

   ■ If you're reading something, say it out loud.

   ■ It might be easier to remember a real book than a digital read according to research from the USA. Apparently, abstract concepts were easier to understand when read on paper; students using only screens had a harder time grasping complex ideas.

   ■ Take a mental picture of your keys on the table, or of information written down.

2 **Don't rely on lists and diaries** – Write it down, read it, visualise it and then leave it at home.

3 **Group items** – It's easier to remember three groups of three than one of nine. Alternatively, invent schoolboy rhymes. For example, 'Our most important organs are our brains, find out why in

---

## CASE STUDY

### GRAHAM: TAKING UP PIANO IN MY FIFTIES

I played brass instruments at school and guitar in bands. But I haven't learned a new instrument for forty-odd years.

A music teacher friend told me it was never too late to learn piano so my wife and I bought ourselves a digital one for Christmas. She's learning it properly – scales and lessons. I tend to just play around a bit like I do on guitar. I'm learning *Imagine* by John Lennon.

Learning is one of the best things for my mental health. Building new pathways in your synapses. It keeps me on a level playing field. About ten years ago I learned French for a similar reason. As an engineer I think I'm a bit what they used to call 'left brain' logical so it's good to learn 'right brain' creative things.

Learning something together and supporting each other is also great for our marriage. We play about an hour a day each, so the only thing we fight about is who is going to use the piano. I suppose we could play one end each!

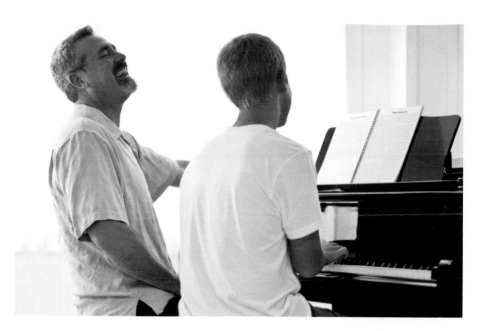

Jim's book from Haynes.' Make up acronyms like the one for the five ways to well-being on page 23.

4 **Say things you need to remember aloud** – to yourself or someone else.

5 **Err...** there is another one. It's really good. No – it's gone.

Crosswords, poker, learning, reading, trying to understand the Large Hadron Collider, trying to understand your TV remote – it's your choice, but the brain is like all muscles: use it or lose it.

## How do you tell if it's dementia and not a bad memory?

It's not easy. My grandad had a brilliant memory but dementia in later life. For a while, his memory for things he was interested in – the betting odds on horses, for example – disguised the deeper problem.

Absent-mindedness is normal when you're busy. Forgetting names is normal.

More worrying is forgetting where you are – especially getting lost in familiar surroundings – or forgetting to put on clothes before going out. Forgetting where you put things is normal: putting them in a totally inappropriate place (like flowers in the fridge) is more worrying. Forgetting a word happens to us all: doing it habitually and substituting other less suitable ones is more worrying.

Anyone can get dementia. Fantasy writer Terry Pratchett had an imagination

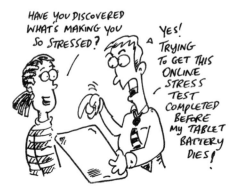

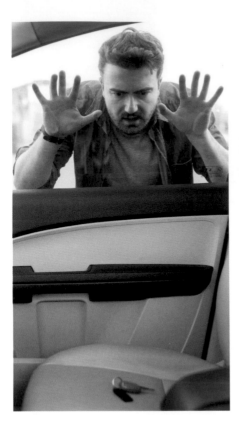

most of us can only wonder at, but he was diagnosed with a form of Alzheimer's disease at the age of 59. Early-onset Alzheimer's like this is very rare (only 5% of cases are in people under 65), but if you're concerned then get advice sooner rather than later.

## Quick Win

### Sniff it out

*Don't neglect your sense of smell. Peppermint, cinnamon and rosemary have all been shown to boost mental alertness. Jasmine and lavender aid relaxation and sleep. Citrus smells may reduce anxiety. What smells do you like?*

## Super sleep

Sleep matters. You spend about a third of your life doing it. Doing it well can make a massive difference to the other two-thirds. These tips may help:

- Keep regular(ish) hours and a regular bedtime routine that helps you wind down
- Avoid stimulants before bed, including exercise, caffeine, fags, booze and heavy meals
- Ideally, use the bed only for sleep, sex and a bit of light reading
- Avoid screens (phones, tablets, laptops etc) for an hour before bed (the blue light keeps you awake)
- Avoid bright light generally – perhaps dim the lights in the rooms you're in before bed as well as the bedroom
- Don't clock-watch (turn the clock away from you) – if you can't sleep, get up and do something boring
- Make sure the bedroom isn't too hot – a degree or so colder than the rest of your home
- Try sleeping alone if you usually sleep with someone (or vice versa)
- Try relaxation techniques such as meditation and yoga
- Try a warm shower before bed
- A small bedtime snack of foods that ease the body into sleep might help – wholegrain cereal, perhaps
- Write down tomorrow's to-do list and other invasive thoughts. Getting them out of your head and onto the page will help put them into perspective and you can quit worrying about them.

# Write a letter

A couple of years ago, a good mate of mine died in his fifties from bowel cancer.

We hadn't seen much of each other for a while. But in our twenties, when we both lived in London, we were, I think, close. Phil was a dry northerner so you could never be entirely sure.

Just before he died, I wrote Phil a letter. A proper letter with a pen. I told him some of the things that I admired in him and thanked him for some of the things he'd done for me. I did it because I thought it was what I'd like someone to do for me, were I in the same situation.

Obviously, I don't know. I've never been in Phil's situation. But I remembered when I had cancer myself – a lot less aggressive than Phil's – and there were a couple of Get Well cards that I hadn't expected from people I didn't really know. One of them, from another dour male, touched me. Even though the religious sentiment didn't mean much to me, I knew it meant a lot to him.

Now, I don't know what Phil made of my letter. It wasn't pub banter. But I do know he read it and I like to think that it meant something to him even if he did think I was a southern softy for sending it.

The selfish point is that it made me feel a bit better. It helped me get a little perspective – not a lot, but enough to feel that life wasn't all a big fat waste of time. Ideally we'd not wait until someone was dying before telling them we like them. But we are blokes so I'm not going to ask for the moon.

Phil once took me potholing and as we were entering the cave he said it was a good idea to look behind you every so often so that you'd recognise the route again on your way out. That wasn't particularly reassuring at the time as I'd foolishly assumed he already knew the route out, but it turned out to be one of the best pieces of advice anyone has ever given me. I still follow it when walking or cycling in the country. When you look behind in this way, you're looking to really see, to fix it in your mind and prepare yourself to see it again in the future. If only – clunking metaphor coming up – we could do that more in life in general: look back occasionally, see the patterns and be wiser.

I sometimes think I learned nothing from having cancer. But looking back, perhaps what I learned was that sending that letter to Phil would be OK.

So go on, take a look behind you. Who do you see on the route you've travelled? Someone who has helped you in your life or meant something? Dad. Brother. Mate. Write them a letter. Email is fine. Illness not necessary. Do it while they're alive.

## Quick Win

**Make a will**

*Sounds morbid, but getting this bit of life admin done will feel like a weight off your shoulders. Guaranteed.*
*It will prompt you to have conversations with those close to you about perhaps the most difficult topic of all, death.*
*Once you've talked about that, you can talk about anything.*

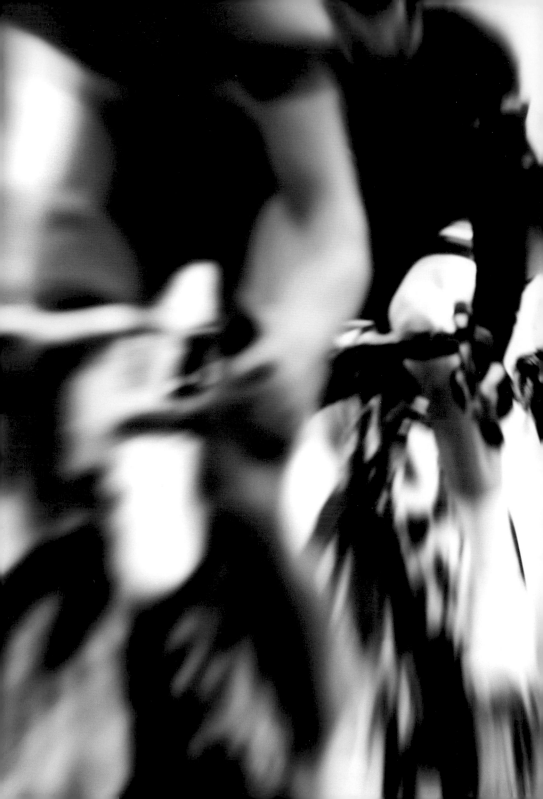

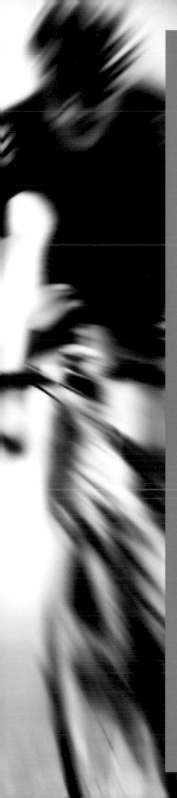

# Chapter 3

# How to be more active

Most men do sport and exercise when they're younger but then let it tail off as careers and families become more important. When this happens, this is the section of the book you need. If you're already a keen exerciser, then this is not really written with you in mind. That doesn't mean you won't find something interesting in it, of course.

The good news is that it's not difficult to get back into the activity game. It needn't even be hard physical work. A physiotherapist once reeled off to me all the men he'd had in his clinic who'd made the same simple and common mistake of assuming that they could exercise in the same way at 40 or 50 as they could at 20. He said the fittest retired guys he knew didn't play sport at all, and some never had – they simply did a gentle 20-minute workout every morning.

# Avoiding the common mistakes

Most physical disability in older age is caused not by lack of muscle or cardiovascular capacity but by lack of flexibility – not being able to stretch or move freely. A short daily workout – the sort of thing you do when warming up for a sport – will stand you in pretty good stead, even if you do little else. Stretching also makes you more resistant to injury as you get older. Just five minutes loosening in the morning will help if you're sitting at a desk much of the day.

Thanks to the likes of Ryan Giggs and the All Blacks, far more men now do activities like yoga and Pilates. Both are accessible, inclusive, and low impact and intensity. Both are great for stability, mobility, muscles and spine. Yoga may have the edge on flexibility and Pilates for strength.

Don't jump straight back into sport. The old saying 'don't play sport to get fit, get fit to play sport' is, alas, true. My physiotherapist's litany of busted knees and broken hearts is the proof.

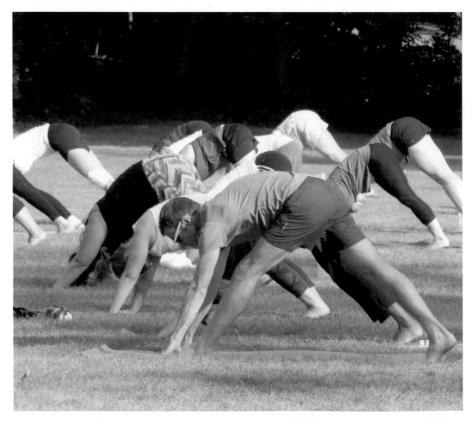

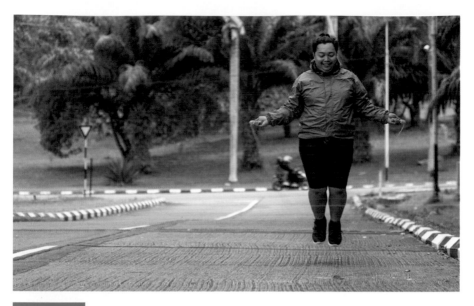

### Remember the good times

*To motivate yourself to exercise, visualise in your mind's eye a positive previous experience – a time when you felt really good: an exhilarating hill walk, a refreshing summer swim, the goal you scored in the Cubs 5-a-side, whatever works.*

## I'm out of condition

If you're out of condition, a little stretching of both your body and your mind is where to start.

You don't have to make big changes. Just build exercise into what you already do. Walk or cycle instead of taking the car. Get off the bus or train a stop early and walk. Use the stairs instead of the lift. All of these little changes really help. In one study, men who averaged at least eight flights of stairs a day enjoyed a 33% lower mortality rate than men who were sedentary. In another, participants saw their chances of premature death reduced by 15% as a result of taking the stairs instead of the lift for just 12 weeks.

It's worth it. A study found that the 20% of the population with the lowest physical fitness levels were twice as likely to die over the next nine years as the 20% with the next-lowest fitness levels. In other words, if you can take yourself from being very unfit to just plain old unfit, you'll make a big difference to your health.

You may need a little tweak to the way you think. Ditch negative thoughts about yourself, your body or your motivation. Perhaps don't even think of this activity as exercise, think of it as going out to play.

If you haven't exercised for several years, are obese or have an existing health problem, check with your GP before starting an exercise programme.

## How do I find the time and money?

Try to make what you do a regular part of your day, not an add-on. For example, should you cycle to and from work every day or go twice a week to the gym? Which are you more likely to do? You have to go to work each day. If you don't cycle you'll have to get there a different way, so why not cycle? The gym is an add-on. You always have a choice and when it's cold or you're tired or your team are on the telly, you can easily choose not to go.

The NHS recommends two and a half hours of moderate intensity exercise a week. Break it down and that's half an hour a day, five days a week. Let's say you swapped the car for cycling into work or even just parked a little further away and got your bike out the boot. You would only have to cycle 15 minutes each way to hit the target. All the rest is gravy.

It needn't be expensive. A lot of us are put off by the idea of wasting money on something we never use. This is true for many gym subscriptions, for example. Modern society has a knack of taking anything that we enjoy and selling it back to us so it's easy to think that you need a lot of gear to enjoy exercise. You don't. My entire bike set-up cost less than £30

> ### Quick Win
> #### *Don't throw money at it*
> *Spending lots of money on kit can deceive you into thinking you've already dealt with the problem. Better to do something free and easy every day than have loads of expensive kitesurfing gear up in the loft.*

including lights. It's less likely to be stolen and, since I'm happy parking it pretty much anywhere, I'm more likely to use it. What's the point of the coolest bike in the world if it stays double-locked in the shed?

As for a cheap gym, there are hundreds of free council-funded, open-air gyms in parks and recs. Free and easy.

> ### Quick Win
> #### *Promise something*
> *Signing up to do a run, walk or swim for charity, or even just promising a mate you'll do the next parkrun, can give you a motivating goal.*

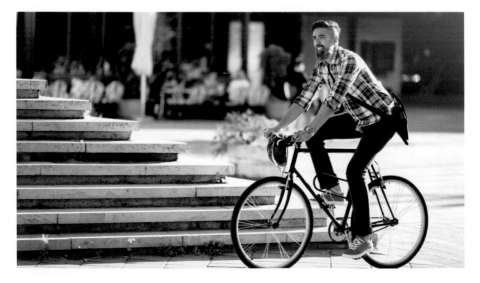

## Best activity to get into?

The simple answer is: whatever you fancy. I've interviewed a lot of starting-over exercisers. There are a couple in this book. For each, there was a moment when they felt that what they were doing made sense – that it fitted in with them, their personalities and their lives. That's what you're looking for, and while somebody else's eureka moment might be interesting, it doesn't mean it will work for you. There's no magic bullet, no one-size-fits-all approach to health. You need to find what works for you.

You can find all sorts of tips and advice about what activity, sport or exercise to do and when. Whatever you choose, the basics boil down to two things:

1   Do something you like doing
2   Don't get injured.

If you manage those two things, you won't go far wrong.

Try standing on one leg for a minute or more. This will give you an idea of how good your core strength is. If you find it very difficult, then do some stretching and specific exercises that will improve your core strength before trying any sports.

The best exercise for avoiding injury is probably swimming. Short of slipping over or picking a fight with the muscular pool attendant, you'll struggle to do yourself any harm in the pool so long as you take it easy. If you are a decent swimmer, you can get just as good a workout in the pool as you can on the track. An hour of jogging at 5 mph or an hour of gentle freestyle both burn about the same number of calories.

Injury lawyers rate rugby, motorbike racing, cycling, cave diving and – would

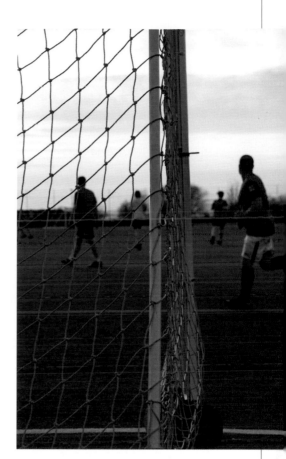

you believe it – cheerleading as the most dangerous sports. Clearly, all contact sports come with an increased risk of injury. So, much as I'd like it not to be so, going back into football or rugby after you've been out of the game for a while may not be your best bet. As every sports fan knows, even the greatest struggle to come back (even The Greatest, Muhammad Ali).

The good news is that non-contact walking versions of many sports now exist. Walking football, walking rugby, walking cricket… you get the idea. Google them. All this is a way of saying that getting active needn't involve running at least not at

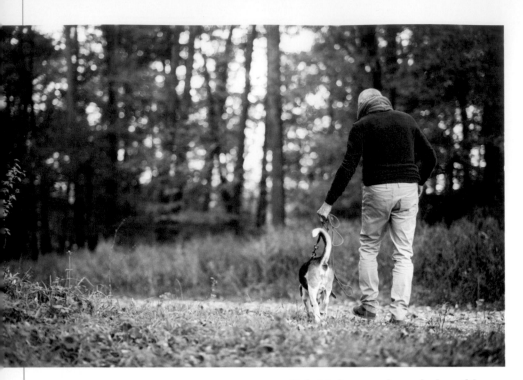

first. In its way, walking can be just as good a fat burner.

Walking also means you're highly unlikely to wind up as one of those people who are forced to give up exercise as a result of injury. The injury risk gets higher the older your body is when you start putting it through its paces. Walkers are far less likely to have exercise-related injuries than runners: a 1–5% risk compared to 20–70%.

> ## Quick Win
>
> ### Build it in
> *Find one enjoyable physical activity you could build into your day. No giggling at the back, I'm thinking about walking, gardening, housework, playing games… but whatever you fancy is good.*

## Point taken: so how do I avoid getting injured?

For those easing back into running or sport, a very useful maxim for ensuring that you remain uninjured is: don't do more today than you will be able to do tomorrow. It's very easy in a burst of enthusiasm to run too far too quickly, with the result that your legs are aching for days afterwards and you don't go out again. It happens all the time to joggers starting over again.

The typical pattern is this. You take it very easy at first, gradually go a little faster and for a little longer each time, and then on the sixth or seventh run you get injured. The reason is that your cardiovascular performance (your heart and lungs, essentially) rises to the task you're setting for it quicker than your muscles and skeleton.

You notice by the third or fourth run that you're already not so breathless as you were the first time. You're really pleased and rightly so. It's a good sign for your lungs, but it doesn't mean that the rest of your body has improved at the same pace – building up effective muscles takes longer. Pushing them to the new limit that you believe your heart and lungs will allow you to will result in injury.

Why? Because the heart and lungs are brilliantly designed organs. They'll get back to something like their best if you work them properly, but your skeleton won't get stronger anything like as quickly. It will always carry the weight of the past 30, 40, 50-odd years and – if you've a bit of a gut – the weight of the present too.

Your body weight can make a big difference. Depending on how you run and on what surface, you're putting three, four, perhaps six times your body weight through your knee with every step. Over a mile, that's 600–800 steps and a lot of weight. So, if you're a big guy to start with, you don't even have to be carrying a spare tyre for your body to start to notice.

That needn't be a problem. Your body will tell you all you need to know, but you need to learn how to listen to it. It's very easy to run through a little aching in the legs, especially when your heart appears to be telling you that it's OK. But that pain is there for a reason, and if you ignore it, you won't be running again for a while. At best, it'll be back to square one; at worst you'll join the hordes who drop out of exercise through injury. A structured programme like the NHS's Couch to 5K will reduce the risk.

Don't run or do sport every day, especially not at first. Often the after-effects are more noticeable two days after exertion than the following morning. Taking your time helps you better get to know your body and how it reacts to what you're putting it through.

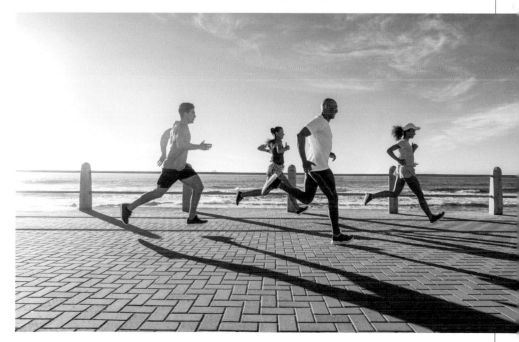

Finally, get the right kit. For most sports this really boils down to decent shoes and – less obviously – the right socks. Most of the rest is fashion.

## Warming up will help, won't it?

Yes. Whatever your chosen exercise, learn how to warm up for it. The normal body temperature is around 37°C, but muscles work best at nearer 38.5°C.

Make sure that you're warming up and warming down the right muscles. This is relatively easy with jogging because walking will do it, but for other sports, find out if you're not sure.

If you're older, will be exercising for longer or are exercising in the morning, warm up for longer. The muscles are tighter after a night in bed. In addition, morning – 10am to be precise – is the peak time for heart attacks, so take it easy.

### Quick Win

**Dance**
*Dance around the house by yourself or with a partner or friend. Play your favourite tune and don't stop moving. Instant physical and emotional therapy.*

Drink about a litre of water for each hour of exercise (including swimming), but don't wait until you're sweating to start. Orange squash is a cheap and simple hypotonic drink for before, during and after exercise.

## How do I know I'm not doing my old heart more harm than good?

For your heart and muscles to get the most from exercise (and keep it safe), the experts reckon that you need to exercise at between 50% and 85% of your maximum heart rate. At 50–70% you're in the so-called 'moderate' intensity zone. At 70–85% you're in the 'vigorous' zone.

The NHS recommend two and a half hours (150 minutes) of moderate intensity exercise or an hour and a quarter (75 minutes) of vigorous intensity exercise a week. In practice, you'll probably do a bit of both.

You can get a pretty good idea of what level of intensity you're exercising at from how your body responds. If you're not so breathless to talk but would struggle to sing, you're probably in the moderate zone. If you're so breathless you struggle to speak (and singing is out), you're probably in the vigorous zone.

If you want to be a bit more scientific about it, use a heart rate monitor. There's all manner of wearable-tech out there. Do you prefer a chest or wrist strap? Does it need to be waterproof or have Bluetooth? A basic one is all you need and they cost no more than a normal watch. This gadget will take account of some of the factors that you might not. Mine showed me how much higher my heart rate was in the morning, for example.

## What do you mean by maximum heart rate?

Your maximum heart rate is 220 minus your age so, if you're 40, your maximum heart rate is 220 – 40 = 180 beats per minute. This makes your moderate zone a pulse of 90–126 beats per minute (50–70% of 180), while your vigorous zone is 126–153 beats per minute (70–85% of 180).

Start out at moderate before you work up to vigorous. A heart rate monitor can help you to stay in the zone. If you're jogging it's easy to follow your heart rate as you exercise. Run until you get out of the

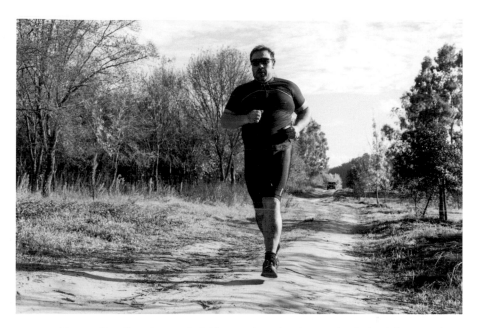

zone and then walk until you're comfortably back in it again. It's less easy – but not impossible – with other activities.

Your effective cardiovascular exercise time is the time you spend in this safe zone, not the time you spend running. Time spent walking in the zone is effective too and puts less strain on your muscles and joints. In other words, joggers starting over can happily spend a lot of the time walking and still get the benefit to the heart. Now, tell me that the body is not beautifully designed.

Time spent below the zone is not doing a great deal for your heart and lungs, although it will still exercise your body. Spend too long above the safe zone and, unless you are an athlete and genuinely fit, you're not doing yourself any favours.

## OK, so I'm in the zone

Build up your routine slowly. A little more – just a minute more or 50 yards further – is fine. You don't even need to do more each time. Just keep going in the right general direction. Do this without getting injured and you may even start to enjoy it. You won't if you're a hobbling wreck after a week.

Finally, if, despite all this, you do get injured, listen to your body. As you get older, the risk of ignoring injuries and pains gets higher. Don't exercise 'through' an injury, rest it, stretch if that helps, and if it doesn't improve, get it checked.

Here's some good advice from Tim Don, the British triathlon and Ironman champion, now in his forties. He suggests would-be triathletes start with swimming.

'It's a great way to get fit and of the three disciplines – running, cycling and swimming – it's the one most people don't do as well,' he says. 'If you do get injured doing one discipline, you can keep your fitness doing the others. Swimming is a great way to recover after an injury or illness – for everyone, not just professional athletes.'

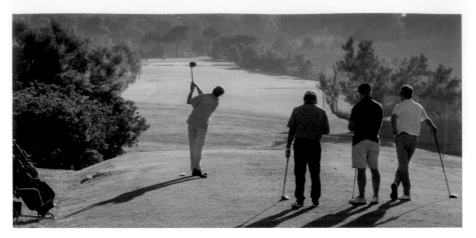

## My strength isn't what it used to be

Men begin to lose muscle mass after about 30. It's estimated that we can lose about 30% over the course of our lives. Muscle loss makes you less mobile and more prone to injury.

No machines or benches are necessary, unless you fancy them. Just a few relaxed repetitions of some simple weights – something relatively light that you can lift without straining or overworking anything – can help remind your body to maintain its muscle.

## Quick Win

### Cheap gym equipment

*Don't like going to the gym or haven't time? Get some equipment at home. There's loads going cheap in charity shops and online. No need for complicated, space-hogging kit. Jump rope, a balance board, cycling pedals, free-weights… they're all small enough to store under the bed. Make sure you know how to use whatever you get hold of.*

## Quick Win

### Old sport

*Try an activity you haven't done for a while – a walk in the park, a swim, ten-pin bowling, golf….*

## Have I left it too late to get good?

Who knows? In his book, *Range*, David Epstein, a journalist interested in sports and science, compares the well-known story of golfer Tiger Woods – swinging a club before he could talk – with the less well-known story of Roger Federer. The tennis star wasn't a prodigy, didn't specialise and played many sports. Mrs Federer was a tennis teacher (which may explain Federer's genetic advantages) but she encouraged him not to take tennis too seriously.

Epstein argues that over-specialisation may make the specialists less effective as time goes on, not more, and create new problems of its own. This suggests that the current way sportsmen (and women) are hothoused – the football academies hoovering up players at ever younger ages, for example – may not be the best way.

But it also says something to the rest of us that might help us to be kinder to ourselves as we age. Epstein reckons his research applies to 'every stage of life'

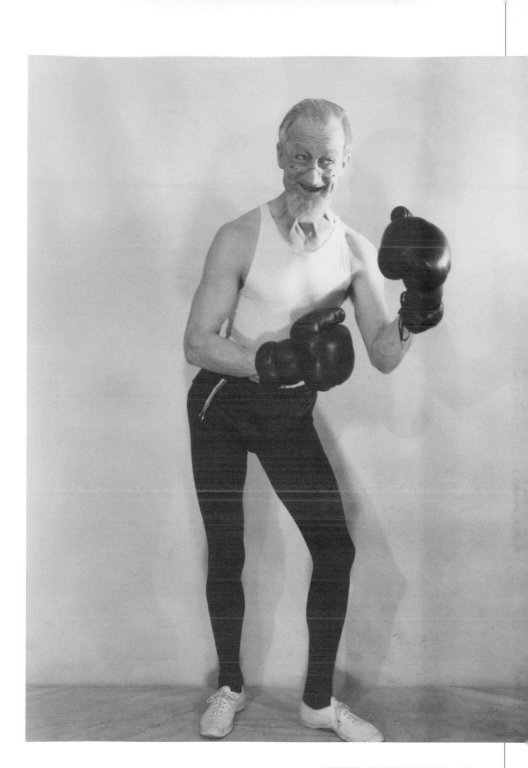

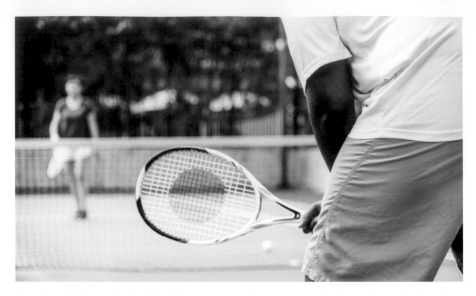

including children, students, 'mid-career professionals' and 'would-be retirees looking for a new vocation'.

To me, this says it's never too late to try what you fancy and you may find that the unique collection of experiences you bring to it may enable you to look at it in a new way. I'm not saying you'll develop a forehand like Roger's but you may find you get the same degree of pleasure from whatever it is that strikes your fancy. You might – and perhaps this remains more important to men than it really should – even be quite good at it.

## Can you exercise too much?

Yes. There is evidence that men who burn 2,000–3,000 calories a week through exercise (equivalent to four to five hours of

jogging or cycling) have lower death rates than both couch potatoes and heavier exercisers. Among other things, over-exercise can result in the production of too much cortisol and boost circulation of free radicals, which can cause cancer.

But how much is too much? There's no hard-and-fast rule. Some say two hours exercise a day, some say burning 4,000 calories a week, some say running 40 miles a week. Suffice to say that if you're exercising at that level you will have looked further afield than this short book for information and advice. All I'd say is: don't put your head in the sand.

The endorphins triggered by exercise can become addictive. So can the attention and admiration of others. Chances are the road to over-exercise will have included some exhilarating highs when you felt like you were at one with the world and 'born' to do whatever you're doing followed more recently by diminishing returns: poorer performance, aching muscles, lower mood and perhaps abnormal heart rate (when not exercising). Get some advice.

> **Quick Win**
>
> ### Never too tired
> *Too exhausted after work to exercise? You might find that exercising when tired will lift your mood and actually reduces fatigue. See if it works for you.*

### Exercise with others

*Combine exercise with your social life by joining a club or team. There are sports opportunities for people of all ages and abilities. Clubs and classes are far more interesting than they used to be – boxercise, boot camp, ballroom (even Bollywood) dancing to name just a few beginning with B. Exercising with your partner is not just good for you both physically, it's great for your relationship too. Quality time together supporting each other - what couple wouldn't benefit from that?*

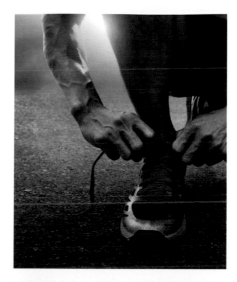

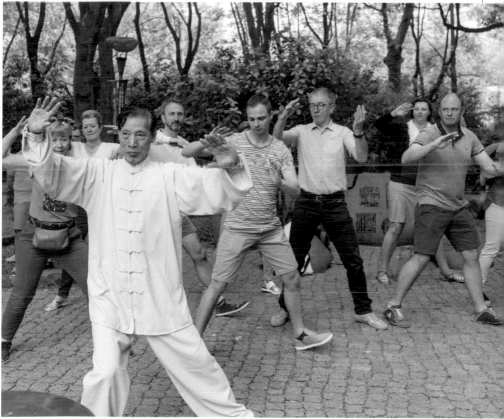

# The world's best exercise? It's a walk-over

Walking is cheap, easy and good for you. It's good for your heart, your mind and your waist, reducing the risk of death, diabetes, depression and dementia.

Two scientists at Harvard Men's Health Watch sifted through the research on walking – some 4,295 articles at the time – and found that walking reduced the risk of both heart problems and of death (during the study period, on average about 11 years) by about a third.

As you'd expect, the greatest benefits were found in men who walked longer distances or walked faster or both. But – and this is great news for everyone – even walking just 5.5 miles per week and at a pace as casual as about 2 miles per hour cuts the risk.

Unlike most forms of exercise, no special arrangements, skills, training or clothes are needed for walking. No warm up, no warm down. It is part of everyday life. Walk to work, walk to the shops, walk the dog, walk to the station. Park your car some way away from where you're going and walk to and from that. Best of all, walk up the stairs. As an activity, this betters even weight lifting.

## Quick Win

**Replace a car journey**
*Replace one regular car journey with a bike ride or walk. It could be to work, the shops, or a leisure or social event. Make it a regular one, though – not that annual visit to relatives.*

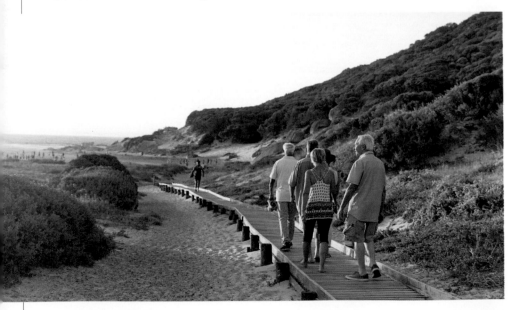

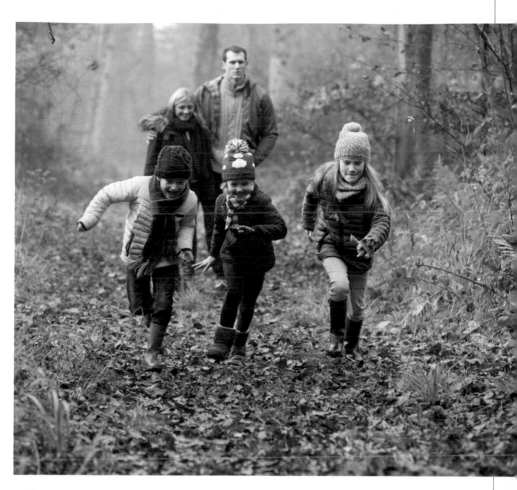

If you can walk faster, so much the better – if you haven't much time or can't walk far, try to walk more briskly to maximise the benefit.

### Boost your walking pace

*Without hurtling around not noticing anyone or anything, increase your regular walking pace. The health benefits are obvious enough, and there is evidence that faster walkers live longer.*

Walking is also a great social activity. It is something you can do with your partner or with a workmate at lunchtime. Or there are umpteen walking groups and clubs out there. Some gallop across fields, others amble around lanes taking in the history. With a bit of luck there's something that takes your fancy near you.

Exercising with others is a great motivator – as is the opportunity to learn something and make new friends. Remember the five ways to well-being that we talked about on page 22–23. A walking group ticks pretty much all the boxes.

### Get a dog

*It's hard to avoid walking when you have a dog. Make sure you genuinely want to look after a pet, though – they need cash and care.*

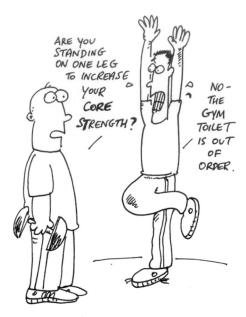

There are all sorts of free pedometer apps for smartphones that will count your steps, time and more. They say aim for 10,000 steps a day. But every little helps.

If walking doesn't sound cool or enough like 'real' exercise, call it low-intensity cardio instead. Walking isn't just slow running. Pro-walkers breeze past the average jogger. Rather, it's a completely different technique: you always have a foot on the ground when walking. That's why it's far lower impact than running. Master it and you have all you need to keep fit for a lifetime. Easy fat-burning. Easy stress reduction.

It's said that most us will walk about 75,000 miles by the time we're 80 – equal to three times around the Earth at the equator. Now that sounds cool.

## Where does the 10,000 steps come from?

Like much health messaging, it's really from thin air. Apparently, it was invented in Japan in the run-up to the 1964 Olympics to market an early pedometer. Useful, though. If you prefer a time target, try three ten-minute walks a day.

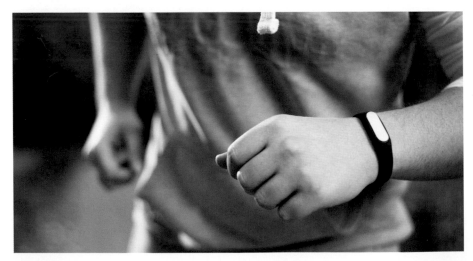

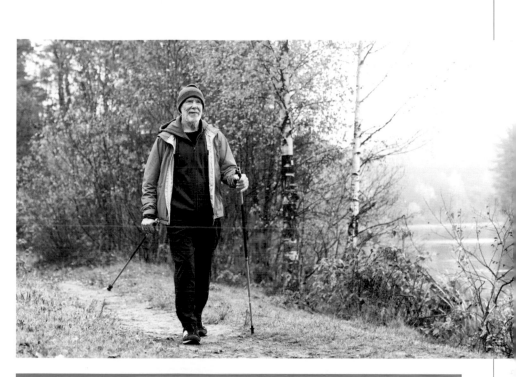

## STEVE: MY WALKING WORKOUT

I didn't really enjoy the gym so I created my own walking routine. I try to do an hour and a half every weekday morning. I got a decent pair of walking boots and found some unused walking poles in my garage.

You don't need the poles, but they incorporate your upper body in the workout and enable you to move more quickly. When it's muddy, they stop you falling.

The total cost is less than £100, which compares to annual gym membership of about £150. But the great thing about walking is that it's in the open air. I walk in all weathers. When you do get a nice day, you savour it all the more.

I enjoy seeing the landscape changing and I've come to appreciate the area in which I live. The woods, the canal. I'm discovering new routes and creating my own.

My walk totals 12,000–13,000 steps and when you add in the usual everyday walking, I'm at about 17,000–20,000 steps a day. I have a pedometer on the wrist which connects to my phone. The app calculates steps, calories, elevation, whether I was faster or slower and so on. I don't think any of this is particularly important but it adds a bit of fun, the way gadgets do.

I feel better and I miss it when I don't do it. I could never say that about the gym.

# Happy heart

The heart is the best bit of kit you've got. It will pump over 100,000 times or more a day without missing a beat. It will speed up automatically when you need more oxygen for exercise and slow down when you need less while sleeping. In return, all it needs for fuel is oxygen, water and a handful of nutrients (available from fruit and vegetables) three or four times a day.

When exercised regularly the heart becomes larger, which means that each beat pumps more blood and thus more oxygen around the body.

Giving up smoking will see your risk of heart disease reduced to that of a non-smoker within three to five years, which is proof of the heart's strength and resilience.

## What's good for the heart?

Five things:

1 Fresh air
2 A balanced diet
3 A healthy weight
4 Regular exercise
5 A relaxed attitude.

Cigarette smoke, pollution, car exhausts and other harmful chemicals in the air make it harder for the heart to do its job. They all cause long-term damage and can trigger heart attacks.

A diet including too much salt and too many of the wrong types of fats can clog up the arteries with a substance called plaque. Again, this can cause long-term damage and trigger heart attacks. There's more on healthy eating in Chapter 4.

The heavier you are, the harder your heart has to work to move you about. The location of the weight also matters. Whereas women get fat around the hips and bum, men tend to get fat around the

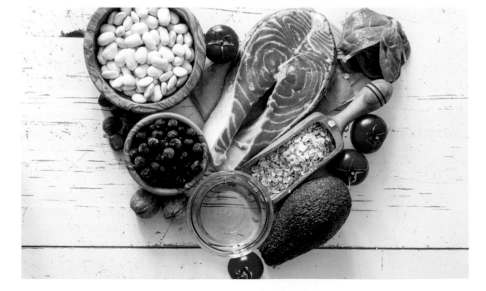

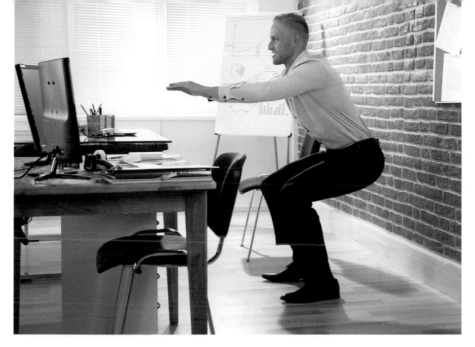

middle, closer to the internal organs like the heart and therefore more likely to damage them. Blood is also more likely to clot in obese people.

To beat at its best over a whole lifetime, the heart needs to work out regularly at different rates, including resting, walking, running and exercising. Men in active occupations have half the risk of heart disease of those in inactive ones. So, if you have a sitting down job you need to get up and get moving to make up for it.

## And a relaxed attitude?

Stress will increase blood pressure. Blood pressure will increase your risk of heart problems, so relax. Nothing's worth having a heart attack for. It's not the end of the

world (unless it is the end of the world, in which case it doesn't matter).

## Are men at more risk of heart disease than women?

Men are more likely to die of heart disease than women. A dicky ticker kills one in seven men compared to one in 12 women. Probably, a tiny bit of this is down to hormones (oestrogen protects) and chromosomes. But mostly it's lifestyle.

The good news is that since the 1960s, death rates from heart disease have gone down by about three-quarters and today about 1.5 million men are living with heart disease in the UK. (There's advice on spotting a heart attack on page 127.)

## So what's bad for the heart?

You probably know most of this already, especially if you've been reading this book. The problem is that the arteries that carry blood from the heart are only as wide as a drinking straw and can easily become blocked up with plaque.

---

**Quick Win**

**'You snooze, you lose'**
*This applies to weight – sleeping better will help you avoid carb-cravings because you're tired.*

---

### Stand up more

*Sitting down all day damages health.
You could:*

- *Walk and talk (on the phone or try walking meetings)*
- *Stand up on public transport (and get off a couple of stops early, too)*
- *Walk to a co-worker's desk and talk instead of messaging*
- *Try a standing desk or work bench.*

- **Family history** – Err… ask your family (more about this on pages 14–15)
- **Exercise** – See Chapter 3
- **Weight** – See the Am I overweight? box on page 68
- **Blood pressure** – There are blood pressure machines in many GPs and pharmacists. Usually free and easy to use. Or you can buy one for about £25
- **Cholesterol levels and diabetes risks** – These are less easy to measure yourself. Talk to your GP. (There is more on diabetes on p88).

Plaque contains calcium and cholesterol and sets like concrete. Plaque increases with age, so the less you produce when you're younger, the better. The main risk factors are: smoking, family history, not enough exercise, being overweight, high blood pressure, high cholesterol and diabetes.

### How do I know if I've got those things?

- **Smoking** – You probably know if you do this. The vast majority of smokers want to quit and we all know why

For anyone over 40 there's an easy solution to all of this. It's called the NHS Health Check. The NHS Health Check is for adults aged 40 to 74. It's designed to spot early signs of stroke, kidney disease, heart disease, type 2 diabetes or dementia. It kicks in at 40 because this is the age at which we begin to be at higher risk of these conditions. If you aren't being treated for any of these conditions already, the NHS should invite you for a check-up every five years. If you think you should have been invited but haven't been, contact your GP and ask for one.

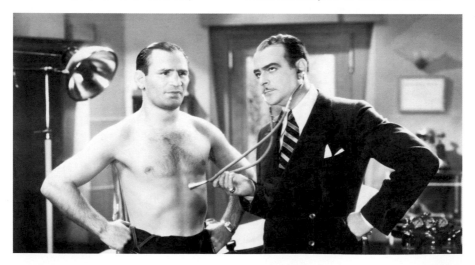

# IAN: RUNNING BACK TO HEALTH

When I was younger, I played a bit of sport; mainly squash and football, but gradually less and less. It didn't matter, I was still young and fit enough to do what I wanted.

I hated cross-country at school so I assumed running wasn't for me. But I got into my forties and went up a trouser size. At a mate's wedding, we all went for a walk and I was knackered. My wife talked me into doing this five-mile race with other parents from our children's school. I thought, fine – I can wing it. But she beat me, in front of all our friends. The shame. That's not happening again, I told myself. Next year, I beat her.

It was a slow burn at the start. I entered races and trained. But I was just running like a kid really. The change came when I entered a marathon and needed to plan for four months of proper training. No more going down the pub afterwards.

Having targets is critical. I need something to work towards. I know exactly how far I've run this week and this year. I never worry about eating or drinking a few more calories. I know I'll burn them off. Obviously I'm fitter. My heart rate is reduced. But the mental health benefits are perhaps greater. A run clears my head. Fresh air, get away from things. Half an hour focused solely on the next step. It's like meditation for me. I also have a whole new group of friends through running.

I know doctors are 'prescribing' running for depression now. Cheaper than drugs. It doesn't work for everyone, but it's great if it does.

If you're starting, do whatever it takes to actually get yourself out there. I'd recommend attainable targets like the Couch to 5K programme. Don't be ashamed to walk. Just don't do something crazy up front. Start simple, perhaps with a group or a mate for encouragement, and build it up.

The barrier to entry is just a pair of shoes. Get a pair that's comfortable. That means trying them on in a shop. Change them when they're worn out. The average life of a running shoe is about 800km (500 miles) – sooner if you're heavier than if you're lighter.

I've been lucky with injuries. I'm small and light and don't put too much strain on my joints. Your musculoskeletal strength improves with time, anyway. You come to understand your own body with time and know what exercises to do if you get a twinge. If you do have an injury, see a sports physio. A GP will probably just tell you to rest, so see a specialist who will be focused on getting you out there again.

There are all sorts of running styles out there. The fact is, we can all run. Our bodies are made for it. We are built to run to outlast our prey, that's our USP as a hunting species.

Running is a big part of my identity. Even when I have a run and it doesn't click, I feel glad I did it afterwards. When it's going well and you're in that flow state, it's just wonderful.

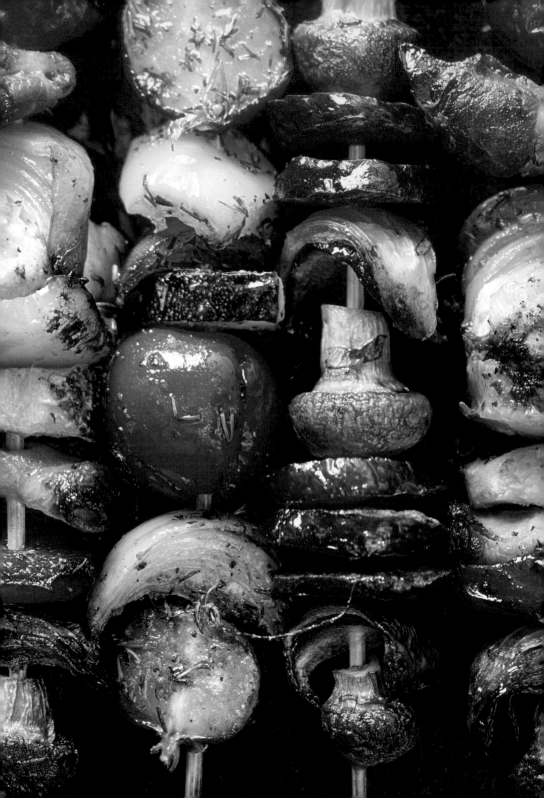

# Chapter 4

# How to eat better easily

Eating and drinking are good things. Very good things. Nothing here about diets. Why? Because diets don't work.

You often hear the phrase 'you are what you eat'. It's not literally true otherwise there'd be a lot of pizzas walking down our high streets. But it is, with the air that you breathe, your main source of fuel. However, unlike with your car, the best fuel is not necessarily the most expensive. Far from it. In fact, eating well is not only good for your mind and body, it's also good for your wallet.

If you want to improve your health easily (and that is the point of this book), finding out more about food and drink, how to put it together, how to choose it and prepare it is one the best things you can do. Your taste-buds will thank you. So will your stomach. Knowing a bit more about good food won't harm your relationships either.

# Diets don't work

If you want to lose weight or eat more healthily, diets with a capital D are generally not your best bet. Diets involving meal replacements, faddy dishes or eating routines usually start well enough but they don't tend to last and they rarely solve the problem. Indeed, many dieters finish up heavier than they started.

There's a fat load of evidence. In 2007, following a review of 31 different studies on this topic, researchers at the University of California concluded that although weight was usually lost during the first six months of a diet, two-thirds of dieters put it back on again – and more – within five years. To make matters worse, yo-yo dieting – where body weight repeatedly rises and falls – can be particularly unhealthy. Losing weight very quickly can actually result in lean tissue being lost rather than fat. Having less lean tissue can reduce your energy needs going forward and encourage weight gain.

Most diets appear to help at first, simply because they force the dieter to think about what he's eating. The thing is they don't deal with the underlying problem: our attitude to food. Men who try to lose weight tend to do so not because they want to get into a size zero dress (although if you do, the advice here still holds) but because they want to feel healthier. Diets that 'forbid' foods and set up 'rules' and 'targets' turn food from a pleasure into a source of shame. Not a healthy feeling at all.

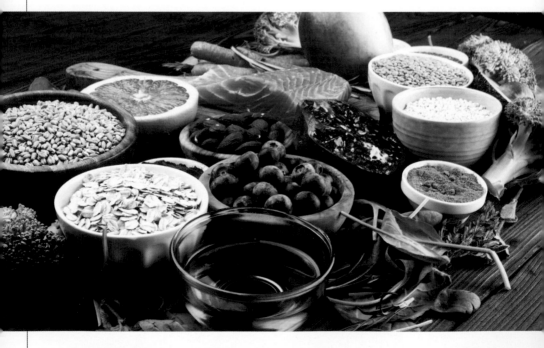

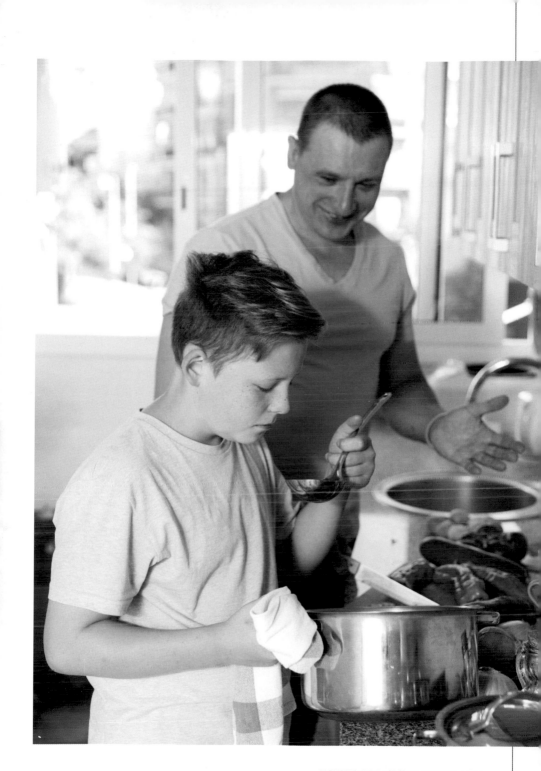

## What do you mean by our 'attitude' to food? I don't have an attitude, I have an appetite

I lived in France for many years. I'm not going to say that French food is better than British food. I'm not even going to say French food is healthier. They love cakes and 'le fast food' just as much as the Brits. But I *am* going to say that the French attitude to eating is healthier.

The French love eating, every single mouthful. I've never met a French person who was on a diet. But it's more than that. They top the league table for time spent eating and drinking, enjoying 2 hours 13 minutes a day at their favourite activity. Eating is life, not a fuelling process. Bottom of the table is the USA – just an hour a day eating and drinking. In the UK, it's 1 hour and 19 minutes. (The international average is about an hour and a half.)

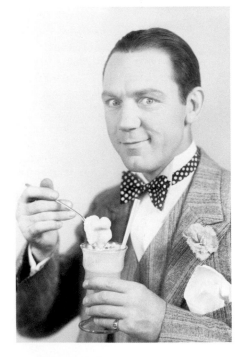

The French eat together. At least one meal a day will be at the table in the company of family or friends, often the evening meal. The British and Americans tend to eat this meal early, wolfing something down before going out or collapsing in front of the TV. In France, people generally eat around 8pm, at the table, meaning that it's often the centrepiece of the evening. You approach your food in a totally different state of mind.

True, French lunch breaks are getting shorter. The pressures of work are global. But it's how you spend the time. Many employers still have canteens where you sit down and eat something decent on a real plate. You may well eat a sandwich, but not at your desk.

The French do snack but there's not a lot of grazing. Why would you spoil your enjoyment of the highlight of the day? As for 'coffee on the go'? No chance. Walking down the street carrying your coffee in a big, paper cup sipping it occasionally through a nasty plastic lid before dumping it still half full? C'est ridicule. Sit down and enjoy your coffee.

It seems counter-intuitive. But seeing eating as an important activity in life – something that is fun, to be shared, to be savoured and to spend time on – may actually mean you eat better.

Let's put it another way, surveys of attitudes and spending suggest that today people of all ages tend to prioritise experiences over things: we'd rather have

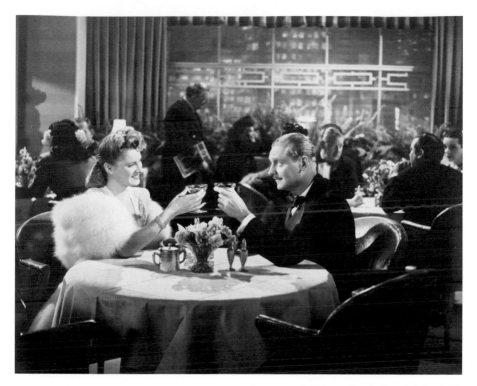

a good night out than buy a new shirt. There's even some serious research suggesting we feel happier spending money on 'doing' rather than on 'having'. If that sounds like you, how about applying that approach to eating? Rather than thinking of foods as things to be eaten, think of meals as experiences to be enjoyed. It might make all the difference.

**Quick Win**

### Save left-overs

*Most of us don't want to waste food. So rather than bin or scoff what's left, freeze it or bung it in the fridge for another meal. Save calories, save cooking. Sounds obvious, but UK households waste about 7 million tonnes of food a year.*

## Does weight matter? I'm fat but fit

I'm sure you are. But even if you have none of the other risk factors for heart disease, research suggests that people who are overweight are still at a greater risk – probably at about 28% greater risk – of a heart attack than someone of 'normal' weight.

Obese people are 40% more likely to die from cancer than those of a healthy weight and are also two to three times more likely to get coronary heart disease.

Adult obesity has pretty much doubled since the early 1990s. Two-thirds of UK men are now overweight or obese. Some politicians and health campaigners talk about an obesity 'epidemic', but while obesity may be up, the number of people who are overweight – about two in five – has stayed pretty much the same.

# Am I overweight?

The standard official measure of how heavy we should be in relation to our height is called the Body Mass Index (or BMI). You can work out your BMI like this:

Weight (in kilograms) / height (in metres) squared

A healthy BMI is anything between 18.5 and 25. Anything below 18.5 is considered underweight. Over 25 is overweight and over 30 is classified as obese. So, generally, if your BMI is over 25, you're overweight and need to act.

It's complicated a bit by ethnicity; Asian men are advised to keep BMI below 23. Plus, because muscle is heavier than fat, some sportsmen – rugby players, for example – can easily have a BMI that, on the face of it, looks too high.

It is easier just to measure your waist. That will give you a good enough guide. Your waist measurement is not your trouser size. Measure at the level of your belly button. If it's over 37 inches (94cm), then you're probably overweight; if it's over 40 inches (102 cm) then you're probably obese.

## BODY MASS INDEX (BMI) CHART

| | | Weight | | | | | | | | | | | | | | | | | | | | |
|---|---|---|---|---|---|---|---|---|---|---|---|---|---|---|---|---|---|---|---|---|---|---|
| | lbs | 90 | 100 | 110 | 120 | 130 | 140 | 150 | 160 | 170 | 180 | 190 | 200 | 210 | 220 | 230 | 240 | 250 | 260 | 270 | 280 | 290 |
| | kgs | 41 | 45 | 50 | 54 | 59 | 64 | 68 | 72 | 77 | 82 | 86 | 91 | 95 | 100 | 104 | 109 | 113 | 118 | 122 | 127 | 132 |
| ft/in | cm | | | | | | | | | | | | | | | | | | | | | |
| 4 ft 8 in | 142.2 | 20 | 22 | 25 | 27 | 29 | 31 | 34 | 36 | 38 | 40 | 43 | 45 | 47 | 49 | 52 | 54 | 56 | 58 | 61 | 63 | 65 |
| 4 ft 9 in | 144.7 | 19 | 22 | 24 | 26 | 28 | 30 | 32 | 35 | 37 | 39 | 41 | 43 | 45 | 48 | 50 | 52 | 54 | 56 | 58 | 61 | 63 |
| 4 ft 10 in | 147.3 | 19 | 21 | 23 | 25 | 27 | 29 | 31 | 33 | 36 | 38 | 40 | 42 | 44 | 46 | 48 | 50 | 52 | 54 | 56 | 59 | 61 |
| 4 ft 11 in | 149.8 | 18 | 20 | 22 | 24 | 26 | 28 | 30 | 32 | 34 | 36 | 38 | 40 | 42 | 44 | 46 | 48 | 51 | 53 | 55 | 57 | 59 |
| 5 ft 0 in | 152.4 | 18 | 20 | 21 | 23 | 25 | 27 | 29 | 31 | 33 | 35 | 37 | 39 | 41 | 43 | 45 | 47 | 49 | 51 | 53 | 55 | 57 |
| 5 ft 1 in | 154.9 | 17 | 19 | 21 | 23 | 25 | 26 | 28 | 30 | 32 | 34 | 36 | 38 | 40 | 42 | 43 | 45 | 47 | 49 | 51 | 53 | 55 |
| 5 ft 2 in | 157.4 | 16 | 18 | 20 | 22 | 24 | 26 | 27 | 29 | 31 | 33 | 35 | 37 | 38 | 40 | 42 | 44 | 46 | 48 | 49 | 51 | 53 |
| 5 ft 3 in | 160.0 | 16 | 18 | 19 | 21 | 23 | 25 | 27 | 28 | 30 | 32 | 34 | 35 | 37 | 39 | 41 | 43 | 44 | 46 | 48 | 50 | 51 |
| 5 ft 4 in | 162.5 | 15 | 17 | 19 | 21 | 22 | 24 | 26 | 27 | 29 | 31 | 33 | 34 | 36 | 38 | 39 | 41 | 43 | 45 | 46 | 48 | 50 |
| 5 ft 5 in | 165.1 | 15 | 17 | 18 | 20 | 22 | 23 | 25 | 27 | 28 | 30 | 32 | 33 | 35 | 37 | 38 | 40 | 42 | 43 | 45 | 47 | 48 |
| 5 ft 6 in | 167.6 | 15 | 16 | 18 | 19 | 21 | 23 | 24 | 26 | 27 | 29 | 31 | 32 | 34 | 36 | 37 | 39 | 40 | 42 | 44 | 45 | 47 |
| 5 ft 7 in | 170.1 | 14 | 16 | 17 | 19 | 20 | 22 | 24 | 25 | 27 | 28 | 30 | 31 | 33 | 34 | 36 | 38 | 39 | 41 | 42 | 44 | 45 |
| 5 ft 8 in | 172.7 | 14 | 15 | 17 | 18 | 20 | 21 | 23 | 24 | 26 | 27 | 29 | 30 | 32 | 34 | 35 | 37 | 38 | 40 | 41 | 43 | 44 |
| 5 ft 9 in | 175.2 | 13 | 15 | 16 | 18 | 19 | 21 | 22 | 24 | 25 | 27 | 28 | 30 | 31 | 33 | 34 | 35 | 37 | 38 | 40 | 41 | 43 |
| 5 ft 10 in | 177.8 | 13 | 14 | 16 | 17 | 19 | 20 | 22 | 23 | 24 | 26 | 27 | 29 | 30 | 32 | 33 | 34 | 36 | 37 | 39 | 40 | 42 |
| 5 ft 11 in | 180.3 | 13 | 14 | 15 | 17 | 18 | 20 | 21 | 22 | 24 | 25 | 27 | 28 | 29 | 31 | 32 | 33 | 35 | 36 | 38 | 39 | 40 |
| 6 ft 0 in | 182.8 | 12 | 14 | 15 | 16 | 18 | 19 | 20 | 22 | 23 | 24 | 26 | 27 | 28 | 30 | 31 | 33 | 34 | 35 | 37 | 38 | 39 |
| 6 ft 1 in | 185.4 | 12 | 13 | 15 | 16 | 17 | 18 | 20 | 21 | 22 | 24 | 25 | 26 | 28 | 29 | 30 | 32 | 33 | 34 | 36 | 37 | 38 |
| 6 ft 2 in | 187.9 | 12 | 13 | 14 | 16 | 17 | 18 | 19 | 21 | 22 | 23 | 24 | 26 | 27 | 28 | 30 | 31 | 32 | 33 | 35 | 36 | 37 |
| 6 ft 3 in | 190.5 | 11 | 13 | 14 | 15 | 16 | 18 | 19 | 20 | 21 | 23 | 24 | 25 | 26 | 28 | 29 | 30 | 31 | 33 | 34 | 35 | 36 |
| 6 ft 4 in | 193.0 | 11 | 12 | 13 | 15 | 16 | 17 | 18 | 19 | 21 | 22 | 23 | 24 | 26 | 27 | 28 | 29 | 30 | 32 | 33 | 34 | 35 |
| 6 ft 5 in | 195.5 | 11 | 12 | 13 | 14 | 15 | 17 | 18 | 19 | 20 | 21 | 23 | 24 | 25 | 26 | 27 | 28 | 30 | 31 | 32 | 33 | 34 |
| 6 ft 6 in | 198.1 | 10 | 12 | 13 | 14 | 15 | 16 | 17 | 18 | 20 | 21 | 22 | 23 | 24 | 25 | 27 | 28 | 29 | 30 | 31 | 32 | 34 |
| 6 ft 7 in | 200.6 | 10 | 11 | 12 | 14 | 15 | 16 | 17 | 18 | 19 | 20 | 21 | 23 | 24 | 25 | 26 | 27 | 28 | 29 | 30 | 32 | 33 |
| 6 ft 8 in | 203.2 | 10 | 11 | 12 | 13 | 14 | 15 | 16 | 18 | 19 | 20 | 21 | 22 | 23 | 24 | 26 | 27 | 28 | 29 | 30 | 31 | 32 |
| 6 ft 9 in | 205.7 | 10 | 11 | 12 | 13 | 14 | 15 | 16 | 17 | 18 | 19 | 20 | 21 | 24 | 24 | 25 | 26 | 27 | 28 | 29 | 30 | 31 |
| 6 ft 10 in | 208.2 | 9 | 10 | 12 | 13 | 14 | 15 | 16 | 17 | 18 | 19 | 20 | 21 | 22 | 23 | 24 | 25 | 26 | 27 | 28 | 29 | 30 |
| 6 ft 11 in | 210.8 | 9 | 10 | 11 | 12 | 13 | 14 | 15 | 16 | 17 | 18 | 19 | 20 | 21 | 22 | 23 | 25 | 26 | 27 | 28 | 29 | 30 |

Underweight     Healthy     Overweight     Obese     Extremely Obese

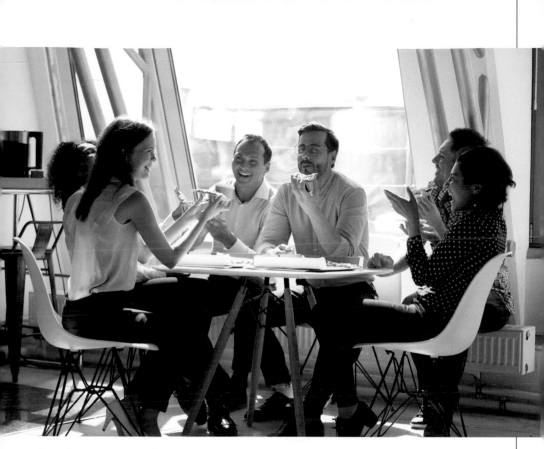

## So what do you do?

Clearly, cutting down on booze and exercising more will help, but if you want to tackle your weight without actually changing what you eat, you need to go slow.

## What do you mean 'go slow'? Take a longer lunch?

That would be a good idea. The point is not to rush your food. To start with, don't even think about *what* you eat, think about *how* you eat. Lots of us stuff our faces in front of the telly, hardly noticing what we're shovelling in.

Take it easy. Look at your food. Chew it. Savour the flavour. Sip some water. You'll enjoy your food more and your body will know that it's actually eating. This is vital, because when it comes to food your brain's a bit slow. It takes it a good 20 minutes to wise up that your stomach is full. This means that if you've been stuffing yourself, you'll have eaten much more than you wanted.

A good rule of thumb that you've eaten too much? The first belch. It's dear old Mother Nature's way of telling you you've had enough. (And, of course, like all mothers, she does it in the most publicly embarrassing way possible.)

You might find you eat spicy food more slowly while the capsaicin in chillies and peppers may help your body's metabolism. (Just don't put your finger in your eye when cooking with chillies – although it might take your mind off food for a while!)

Once you're eating more slowly, you'll taste your food better. So the smart next step might be to choose the tastiest version of it.

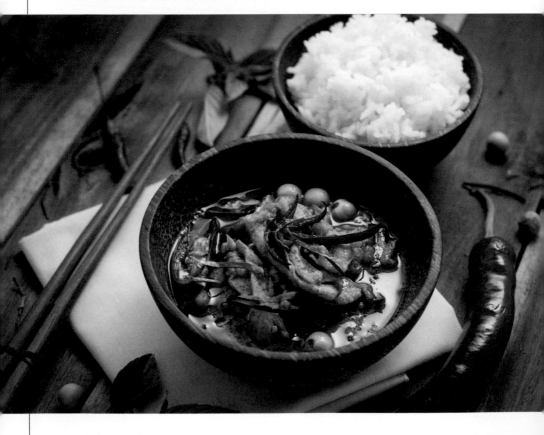

## I like the sound of 'tasty'

The carrot that tastes most like a carrot will probably be the one you've pulled out of the ground yourself, or bought from a local source, rather than the one that was picked weeks ago and has since been flown round the world, sliced up, salted, sugared and tinned. The fresher version is probably also the most nutritious version with the most vitamins.

There's nothing in principle wrong with tinned food. It's handy and easy to use. But the more factories and other processing places your food has been through, the more likely it is to have had sugars, salt and fats added.

Baked beans are a good example of the problem with processing. The beans themselves are very good for you but in the tins we buy they're often pumped up with salt and sugar.

It's important to check the labels on tinned and other processed foods. You'll be surprised how much salt, sugar and other stuff is added. Try to choose the versions with the least salt and sugar. The red, amber and green traffic-light flashes on food labels can help you. As with traffic lights on the road, red and amber mean stop and green means proceed with caution. Obviously, you want as much green as possible.

Ready meals and convenience pre-packed options often have hidden salts and sugar too. So don't buy a chicken meal; buy a chicken.

That is not to say that all fresh food is all that fresh. If the item has been flown from the other side of the world then it's likely to be less fresh than something produced down the road. Check out the countries of origin of fruit and veg and buy local produce whenever you can.

Apart from the reduction in nutrients, processed foods (and fast foods like burgers and fries) have a high energy density. That means that each mouthful contains a lot of calories. Human beings have evolved over thousands of years to guess how much we need to eat by the size of a portion, but an ordinary-looking

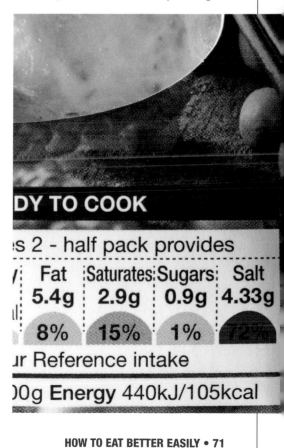

DY TO COOK

s 2 - half pack provides

| | Fat | Saturates | Sugars | Salt |
|---|---|---|---|---|
| | 5.4g | 2.9g | 0.9g | 4.33g |
| | 8% | 15% | 1% | 72% |

ur Reference intake

0g Energy 440kJ/105kcal

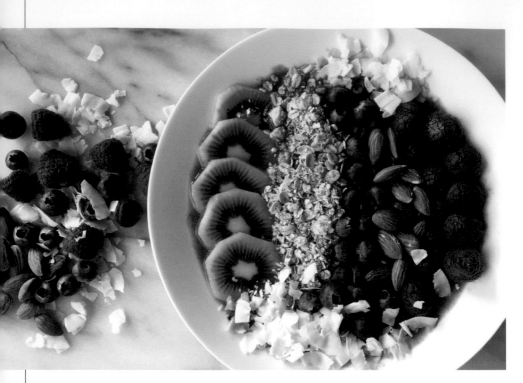

portion of a high-density food can contain double the calories your body expects. If you also eat quickly, you can see how the calories can mount up.

Worst of all, you can become dependent on the sweet, salty, fatty tastes because they give you an instant sugar hit. In tests, rats that become used to this sort of food get the shakes when they're deprived of it. Trouble is, the hit soon wears off and you're starving again. Now, if only you'd eaten more slowly in the first place. Just like mamma used to say.

## Are you saying the way we eat today is unnatural?

Well, let's put it this way, the foods we eat now are very different from those we've eaten in the past. Humans like us have been on Earth for at least 200,000 years and 'homo' species very similar to us have

been around for at least two million years. So, relatively speaking, the cultivation of crops only began yesterday and the processing of food an hour ago.

That's why you hear people going on about the raw food diet or the caveman diet. Sure, they're trying to sell diet books, but the basic theory is sound. For most of our time on this planet, we've been eating what we could hunt and what we could gather from the landscape around us. That means a diet of mainly fruit, nuts, vegetables and meat.

This is not to say that the meat would be much like today's meat. The meat on a hunted animal is different from the flab on a factory-farmed one that has never seen daylight or walked more than a yard or two. Lean meat, free range, organic or game is closer to what you're after.

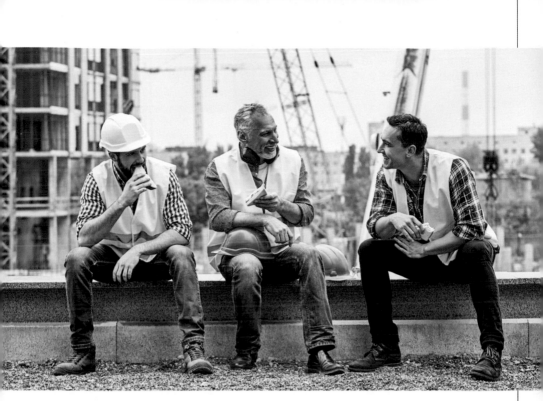

## So, it's OK to eat meat?

That's up to you. (Check out the section on page 82: Should I stop eating meat?) But from a health point of view, good quality meat is fine in moderation (around twice a week).

## Should you take supplements?

For most men, most of the time, the answer is probably no. It's best to get all your nutrients from your diet, if possible.

The one exception to this is perhaps vitamin D.

Vitamin D, which is vital to bone health, is found in a few foods (oily fish, red meat, liver and egg yolks) and is also added to some processed food including spreads and cereals but not, in the UK, dairy milk. However, the main source of vitamin D is sunlight and the NHS reckon that most of us in the UK don't get enough between October and early March.

If you want to explore particular supplements, check the safe dose and whether the supplement is really 'bioavailable'. It is quite possible to take too much of some vitamins and minerals. Equally, it is quite possible that your supplement will just pass through your body, providing you with little except a depleted bank account.

It goes without saying that you shouldn't buy magic muscle pills from that bloke in the changing room of the gym with the staring eyes.

### Quick Win

**Brushing teeth after meals**
*Wait half an hour, especially if you've eaten something fairly acidic. Rinse with water in the meantime, if you want.*

## If cereals are new in our diet, does that mean they're bad for me?

Not at all, but you should try to get the version of the cereal or crop that's closest to nature. Opt for unrefined carbs. That means oats, wholegrain bread, brown or wild rice and brown pasta.

If you're having trouble eating five portions of fruit and veg a day, replace one serving of refined carbs or cereals with one of vegetables.

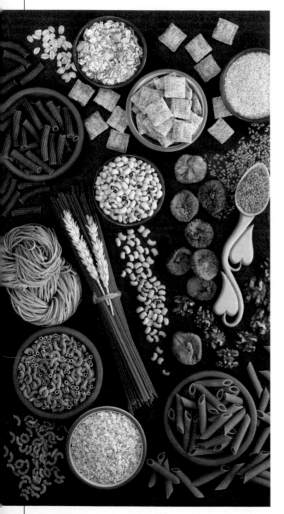

## You could cut down on carbs just by skipping breakfast

You could, but are you craving something mid-morning as your body cries out for nutrients?

I'm a big fan of breakfast but the idea that it's the most important meal of the day is probably misleading. Research suggesting that breakfast-eaters are healthier than non-breakfasters probably says more about the people than the meal. That is to say that, as a rule, people who eat breakfast probably eat more healthily generally than those who don't. So provided you eat well the rest of the time, skipping breakfast is of itself probably not bad for you.

## I'm still piling on the pounds

Here is the easiest dietary change that I've come across. I won't call it a diet because it doesn't ask you to change anything.

Prepare and cook your food in the same way and in the same quantity as usual but only serve half. Put the rest in the freezer compartment for another time. You'll get all your usual nutrients, just fewer calories. If you can do it, it will work. Halving your evening meal will see you losing about two pounds a week. Drink a glass of water ten minutes before you eat to take the edge off your appetite.

That's it.

### Quick Win

**Keep a food diary**
*Note what you eat for a week or a month. Knowing you're doing this promotes healthier choices in the first place and seeing it in black and white afterwards makes it easier to spot the changes you need to make.*

# Foods in focus

## SALT

We eat salt:

- Naturally in food
- Added by manufacturers in food processing
- Added by us when cooking or eating.

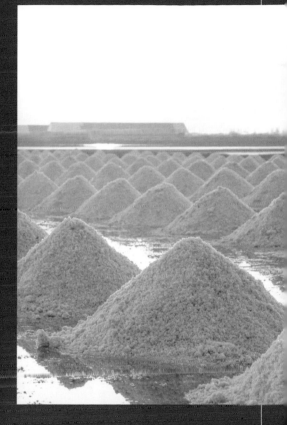

The recommended maximum per day from all three sources is one teaspoon (6g). Not a lot.

About three-fifths of salt in the average diet comes from food processing, so on labels check the amount of sodium per 100g. (You'll remember from school science that the chemical name for salt is sodium chloride. What you won't know is that 6g of salt, which is already not a lot, equals just 2.4g of sodium.) Over 1.5g of sodium per 100g is a lot and best avoided. Aim for 0.3g per 100g maximum or 'no added salt'.

Try not to add any salt at the table and go easy when cooking.

---

**Quick Win**

### Improve sauces and dressings

*Mix sauces and dressings with your favourite milk to reduce salt and calories. They go further and often taste better. Ready-meal sauce sachets are often enormous. Use some and save the rest.*

**Quick Win**

### Herby rides again

*Explore herbs and spices – a great healthy alternative to salt for adding flavour to food.*

# SUGAR

The health impact of too much sugar in our diet has become so clear over the last decade that in 2015, Public Health England halved its guidelines on sugar. The maximum recommended amount of so-called free sugars is now equal to about seven cubes of sugar (30g) a day. So don't add sugar if you can help it.

All the sugar added to bread, cereals, biscuits, ready meals, cakes, drinks, fizzy drinks and all the other processed food we eat adds up to seven sugar cubes quite quickly. Check food labels for added sugars and those found naturally in honey, syrups and fruit juice (even unsweetened).

Look for the 'Carbohydrates (of which sugars)' figure on the packet. Even food marked low sugar can contain up to 5g of sugars per 100g.

Sugar can also be found hidden in the list of ingredients. Corn syrup and any ingredients ending in -ose are all sugars. Examples include sucrose, glucose and fructose. Probably best avoided if they're near the top of the ingredients list.

No need to count the sugars found naturally in whole fruit and vegetables (and in milk and milk products like plain yoghurt). They're OK in moderation.

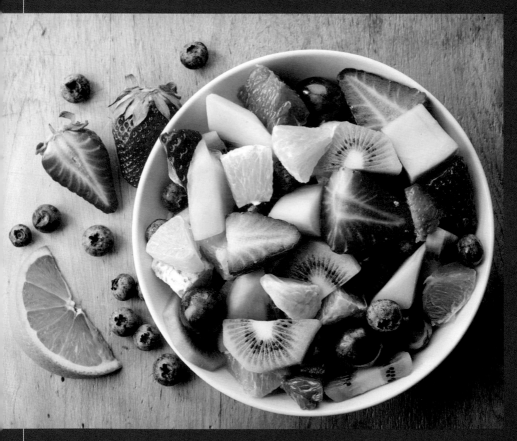

## ARE YOU SAYING AN ORANGE IS OK BUT ORANGE JUICE ISN'T?

The sugar behaves differently. In a whole fruit (or dried fruit) the sugar is still within the fruit. The juicing process changes this. You could say it frees the sugars up. As a result they're absorbed into the body in much the same way as a spoonful of sugar, the unhealthy way.

Choose whole fruit over shop-bought juices or smoothies. Or make your own smoothie, perhaps including some veg to reduce the sugar content.

## IS SUGAR ADDICTIVE?

Carbohydrates affect mood by triggering the release of feel-good brain chemicals such as serotonin. This can make you crave similar foods. However, these effects are not as addictive as, for example, nicotine or alcohol. The craving we often have for something sweet will pass.

Scientists have also found stress hormone receptors within the taste buds that detect sweetness, which may explain why we turn to sweet foods when stressed.

If you crave something sweet, distract yourself. Exercise will do this best – a walk or run – as it will burn off the effects of stress and also curb the cravings, but anything that keeps you absorbed will help. If you can't get away, drink water or herbal tea.

## CHOOSE LOW-SUGAR ALTERNATIVES?

Choose naturally low-sugar products, rather than those that use artificial sweeteners.

It seems like a no-brainer to choose the diet version of your favourite soda – same sweet taste, no sugar. But, if

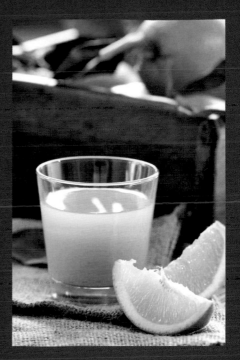

anything, the sugar sensation in your mouth is even stronger than with real sugar, which may increase cravings. Some say it even tricks your body into thinking that it is consuming a lot of sugar and so should lay some down as fat. Certainly, diet soda drinkers appear more likely to be overweight and more at risk of diabetes.

### Quick Win

**Delay dessert**
*You might find the urge for something sweet passes and you want one less. If the craving won't quite go, share desserts (works as well at home as in the restaurant). Or put a healthy dessert out at the start of the meal (fruit, plain yoghurt) rather than choosing one later when your taste buds might be more excited.*

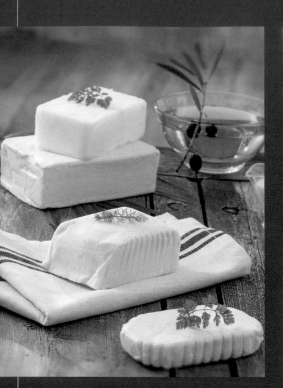

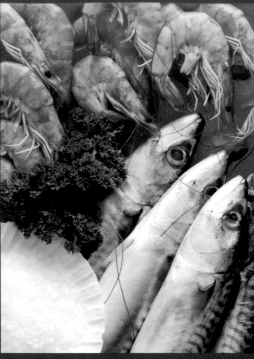

## FATS

There are several types of fat, including trans fats (best avoided), saturated fats (which we need a little of) and unsaturated fats.

Unsaturated fats are the most healthy and can reduce cholesterol. As well as oily (or fatty) fish, sources include (unsalted) nuts; seeds; oils such as sunflower, rapeseed and olive; and avocados.

All fats, good and bad, are high in calories – 9 calories per gram (compared to 4 calories per gram for carbs and protein).

### WHAT ARE TRANS FATS?

They're an industrial product created when vegetable oils are converted into something solid and 'spreadable'. They give products a realistic feel in your mouth, as well as a longer shelf life.

Sounds harmless, but worldwide, trans fats are responsible for half a million deaths per year according to the World Health Organisation. The UK food industry is trying to wean itself off them. It is said trans fats are not used in food processed here, but are still found in food from abroad.

Look out for them in margarines, baked products, cereals, fried foods, sweets, chocolate products, spreads, soups, salad dressings, snacks, ice cream and frozen breaded products. There's no legal requirement to label trans fats specifically. Look for words like 'hydrogenated', 'shortening' and, of course, 'trans' on the food labels.

## YOU SAY FATTY FISH IS GOOD FOR YOU

The fats in oily fish, such as omega-3, are called essential fatty acids. They're 'essential' because the body can't make them itself. We need to get them from our diet.

Omega-3 tops the list of nutrients for the brain. They're found in salmon, trout, mackerel, herring, sardines, pilchards, whitebait, tuna and anchovies. Tinned fish is fine (and easy to buy, store and eat). The tinned varieties of these fish will, in general (with the exception of tuna) contain decent levels of healthy fats.

Shellfish, like mussels, oysters, carb and squid, also contain omega-3. Shellfish are also high in zinc, which helps male fertility.

White fish, like cod, haddock, plaice and sea bass, while good for you because they're low in unhealthy fats, don't contain as many omega-3s. If you fancy some fish, poach, bake or grill it rather than deep frying it. Keep fish and chips as an occasional treat.

The NHS recommends at least two portions of fish a week, including one of oily fish. (However, don't eat more than four portions of oily fish a week as they can contain low levels of pollutants like mercury, especially from fish near the top of the food chain like tuna, swordfish or shark.)

Omega-3 is also found in meat. Grass-fed meat and dairy products are better choices than grain-fed ones.

## ANTIOXIDANTS

Antioxidants cancel out the cell-damaging effects of so-called free radicals.

Free radicals are atoms, molecules or ions that have a spare electron and so are looking around desperately for other free electrons to bond with. It is better that they bond with an antioxidant because bonding with your DNA could cause cancer. Imagine a great big dance floor, last dance at the prom: if those free radicals don't have an antioxidant to dance with, they're going to be angry. That's the theory anyway.

Antioxidants include vitamins C and E, selenium, and carotenoids, such as beta-carotene and lycopene. They're common in fruit and veg. See the '15 favourite foods for men' box, overleaf, for some good sources.

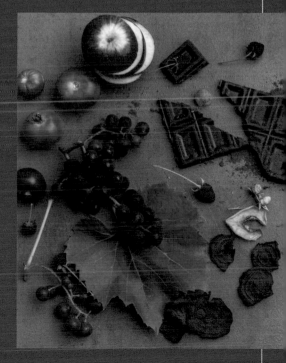

# 15 FAVOURITE FOODS FOR MEN

1  **Broccoli** – Beta-carotene, omega-3, vitamins C and E plus B vitamins, 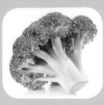 calcium, iron and zinc. There's no such thing as a superfood, but broccoli comes pretty close.

2  **Carrots** – The richest source of beta-carotene (all orange and red veg are a good source; perhaps try  sweet potato if you don't like carrots).

3  **Citrus fruits and pineapple** – Vitamin C (pineapple juice is not dissimilar to stomach acid, so not great for your teeth).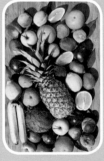

4  **Garlic** – A natural antibiotic, the king of healing foods is good for cholesterol 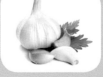 and blood pressure (for best results, eat fresh garlic as soon as possible after chopping, but pastes are easier and pickled garlic is a less-smelly alternative).

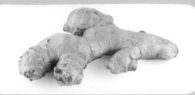

5  **Ginger** – Full of good stuff, ginger is a natural prevention for travel sickness and nausea. (By the way, both garlic and ginger are said to be good for your sex drive.)

6  **Walnuts** – Top non-animal source of omega-3 fatty acids and a great source of antioxidants. 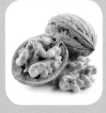 (Also high in antioxidants are pecans, chestnuts, peanuts and pistachios. Most nuts are good for you but beware of calories and added salt and sugar.)

7  **Sunflower seeds** – Top seed for antioxidants, especially vitamin E (two tablespoons (28 g) daily will double most people's vitamin E intake). 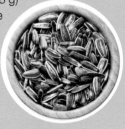 Other antioxidising seeds include poppy seed, linseed, sesame seed and pine kernel. Pumpkin seeds are also high in zinc and magnesium and may be good for your prostate, sperm quality and sex drive.

**8  Chilli** – High in vitamin C and beta-carotene, chilli also boosts calorie burning.

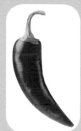

**9  Tea** – High in antioxidants called flavonoids. Choose lighter tea (oolong, green, jasmin) for maximum benefits.

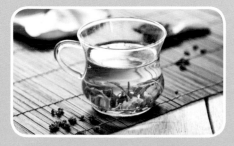

**10 Dark chocolate** – Also high in flavonoids plus iron, magnesium and zinc (only a square a day, but you knew that already).

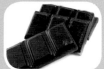

**11 Avocado** – Another great source of antioxidants and omega-3s, but again, watch the calories.

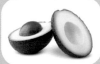

**12 Banana** – A great high-fibre source of the antioxidant dopamine and of potassium,

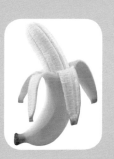

which helps regulate blood pressure. Try plantain too.

**13 Tomato sauce** – A great source of lycopene. Sun-dried tomatoes and tomato puree contain more than fresh tomatoes because cooking frees the lycopene, making it easier for the body to absorb. Lycopene gives red fruit its colour meaning it's also found in guava, pink grapefruit, watermelon and papaya.

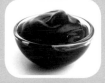

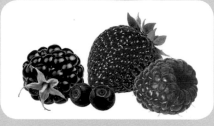

**14 Berries** – Antioxidants again. Cheaper and easier to use if bought frozen.

**15 Oats** – Always 'whole' (unrefined), so compared with other cereals they always retain their natural nutrients including B vitamins, minerals including iron and zinc, antioxidants and fibre.

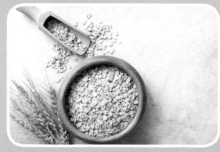

# Should I stop eating meat?

The World Health Organisation classifies red meat and processed meat as cancer-causing. That doesn't mean they're as dangerous as tobacco or asbestos but it does mean you need to keep a close eye on how much you're eating.

It's hard to quantify the risk exactly, but the NHS advises no more than 70g a day of red and processed meat. That's not a lot. The NHS reckon that a cooked breakfast containing two typical British sausages and two rashers of bacon is equivalent to 130g.

Red meat includes beef, lamb, pork and similar meats (not chicken, turkey or game). Processed meat includes sausages, bacon, ham and deli meats. Of the two, processed meat carries probably the higher risk – the World Cancer Research Fund advise eating 'little, if any, processed meat'.

Having said all that, meat contains vital protein, iron, zinc, vitamin B12 and other nutrients that we all need to include in our diet.

Health-wise there's not much difference between a low-meat and no-meat diet. However, most people do not become vegan or vegetarian for health reasons. There has long been concern about animal welfare. In the drive for more and more, cheaper and cheaper meat, it's the animals that suffer.

Recently, an arguably even bigger concern has emerged: the devastating impact on the environment and climate of livestock farming. Meat provides about 18% of human calories but uses 80% of the world's farmland, while even the most environmentally friendly beef products produce six times the global emissions of the equivalent plant protein. Meat production has snowballed to four or five times the level it was in the 1960s. As the world's population continues to grow, the current model is unsustainable.

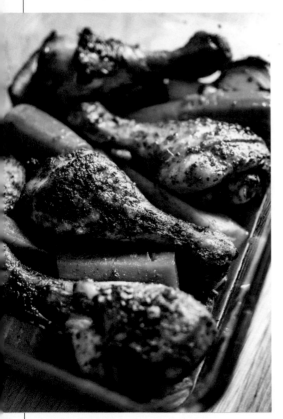

## Quick Win

### Find a new vegetable
*Try some veg that you think you don't like. Or even a vegetarian or vegan meal. Bonus points if you can cook it.*

### Try protein snacks

*A small carbohydrate snack (biscuits, pretzels, etc.) may only spike your blood sugar and leave you craving more carbs. Try a protein snack (nuts, seeds, yoghurt or cheese). How about slices of apple with a spoonful of peanut butter?*

## What about my protein? Do I have to eat tofu?

There are many alternative sources of protein including fish, lentils, chickpeas, other beans and pulses, nuts and seeds, quinoa, mushrooms and cheese (especially cottage cheese, which is lower in fat and contains more protein per calorie). Broccoli and peas both contain protein. So do eggs and dairy products like milk and yoghurt.

Edamame beans are very trendy – they're baby soya beans.

## What about other nutrients like B12?

There are some nutrients that are difficult to get without some meat in your diet. These include:

- **Vitamin B12** – Important for brain function and energy, B12 is pretty much only found in animal-sourced food
- **Creatine and carnosine** – Important for muscle (including the brain) but only occurs naturally in animal tissue
- **DHA (docosahexaenoic acid)** – Important for the brain and found mostly in fish
- **Iron** – Although the iron in red meat is particularly well-absorbed by the body, there are many vegetarian alternatives including beans, pulses, nuts, seeds, grain and certain fruits and vegetables.

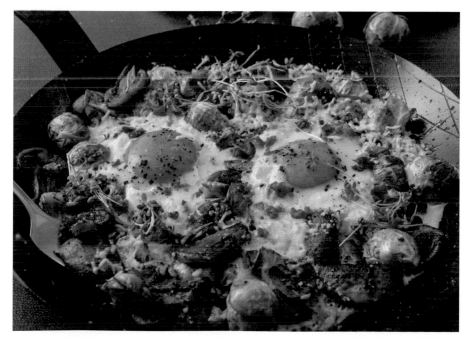

Supplements are available for most of these nutrients if you need them. Many vegans and vegetarians take B12, for example. Cereals and non-dairy milk can be fortified with B12.

On the positive side, a healthy vegan or vegetarian diet can reduce the risk of weight gain, heart disease and some cancers. About one in eight Brits now say they are vegetarian or vegan, with about a third of the population reducing their meat intake.

## But I like eating meat

You're in luck as meat substitutes are now everywhere. The Greggs vegan sausage roll (made from Quorn) is perhaps the best known in the UK, but a lot of burger chains and even Wetherspoons are getting in on the act.

Currently, the 'meat analogues', as food scientists apparently call them, include tofu (made from soya), tempeh (from fermented soya) and seitan (from wheat gluten) but the race now is to create the look and feel of meat: the 'blood', the fibrous texture. The big food corporations are on board and the next few years will see meat analogues on plates across the world. These products should be far less environmentally damaging than the meats they are designed to replace. I don't doubt many of them will be very tasty but the thing to remember is that all these are highly processed foods with thickeners, emulsifiers, sugar and salt. 'Whole' foods they ain't.

The holy grail is to create meat from animal cells in the laboratory: real meat 'grown' without harming the environment or living animals. We have the technology but not yet at the price of a Big Mac. When the world's first lab-grown burger

appeared in 2013, it cost $330,000. Very nice with fries.

## Is soya 'bad' for men?

Soya (or 'soy' in the USA) is a great source of plant-based protein and nutrients. It may help lower cholesterol. But because it contains compounds that are similar to the female hormone, oestrogen, questions have been asked about the impact of soya on the male hormone, testosterone. The research suggests this is a big fat myth: it makes no difference. Eating soya won't reduce your testosterone levels. In fact, it may even protect a little against prostate cancer. Good news if you enjoy soya milk on your cereal.

There is, however, a good reason to go easy on the soy source: it's not the soya beans, it's the high salt content. (If you can, choose naturally fermented soy sauce; the cheaper chemically fermented one may contain toxic compounds called chloropropanols.)

---

### Vegan, veggie or what?

- ■ **Vegan** – Neither eat nor use animal products or by-products.
- ■ **Vegetarian** – May eat animal by-products, so a lacto vegetarian eats dairy, an ovo vegetarian eats eggs and a lacto-ovo vegetarian eats both dairy and eggs.
- ■ **Pescatarian** – Avoid all meat except fish and seafood (so not strictly a form of vegetarianism). Many are concerned that the way we catch and farm fish is unsustainable too.
- ■ **Flexitarian** – Veggie diet with occasional meat, so definitely not a form of vegetarianism.

# Bread alone

Look at the ingredients in a loaf of bread and you may be a little surprised. Some breads are high in salt, some in fat, some in sugar, some in the lot. Often, these loaves have healthy-looking images on the packaging, all ears of grain and seeds. There is also a massive variation in calories, with some breads having twice as many per slice as others. Worth checking the labels on your favourite loaf.

The healthiest breads will be made from wholegrains, which retain all the natural nutrients including B vitamins, folic acid, iron, selenium, magnesium and fibre. Look for the word 'whole' on the ingredient list. If it ain't there, it ain't wholegrain, regardless of how many healthy descriptions like 'multigrain' or '100% wheat' or 'unbleached flour' are plastered over the packaging.

Processed bread, which is usually white, removes the bran and germ from the wholegrain. It has a longer shelf life and is easier to digest but has none of the good stuff: no fibre or vitamins or minerals. These are often added back in the manufacturing process, but added vitamins and minerals are not as easily absorbed by your body as the real thing in real grains. Too much white bread can also increase the risk of diabetes, heart disease and obesity.

Even if you do find the word 'whole' on your ingredients list, look out for added preservatives, salt and sugar.

Want to be sure of your bread? Bake it yourself. It's fun. Slightly messy fun. You tend to get absorbed in what you're doing, which makes it good for mental health. A bread-making machine can simplify it if you don't have the time or inclination but fancy a bread you know to be fresh and full of fine stuff.

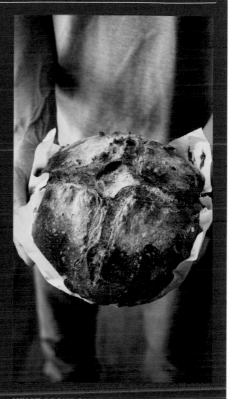

## WHAT ABOUT GLUTEN?

Gluten is the new demon of the everyday diet. Unless you have celiac disease or a genuine gluten intolerance, gluten is fine to eat. Avoid gluten for no good reason and you may find yourself missing out on wholegrains. Research suggests that while eating gluten doesn't cause heart disease, avoiding wholegrains so as to avoid gluten might.

Some people have an intolerance to wheat rather than gluten. If you think that bread or similar products are making you feel bloated or uncomfortable, get it checked out by a doctor rather than just assuming you have a gluten intolerance.

# Gut feeling

Your gut is a major ecosystem. It apparently contains more than 50 trillion microbes from over 1,000 different species. Gulp. Good gut health helps digestion and also your immune system and mood.

As ever, it's high-fibre, whole foods, fruit and veg that you need to eat for good gut health. They help so-called good gut bacteria (probiotics) to thrive, while antibiotics and processed foods do the opposite. Fermented foods are particularly rich in probiotics and will give your gut a helping hand. Types of common fermented foods include:

- Kefir (fermented milk)
- Sauerkraut (raw cabbage)
- Gherkins (pickled cucumbers)
- Tempeh (soya beans, Indonesian)
- Natto (soya beans, Japanese)
- Some types of cheese (including cottage cheese and ricotta)
- Kombucha (tea)
- Miso (soya beans)
- Kimchi (cabbage and radish, Korean)
- Yoghurt (fermented milk, fewer healthy bacteria and less protein than kefir)
- Sourdough bread
- Olives

Of course, not all fermented products are friends of your gut. Salami (which is fermented meat, usually pork) and beer and wine should be consumed in moderation.

## How do I know if I have poor gut health?

Your gut will tell you. Bloating, diarrhoea, constipation, cramps and gas may all be signs. If symptoms like these persist, you may have irritable bowel syndrome (IBS). This affects about 11% of men.

Don't just rely on over-the-counter treatments. It's important to see your GP to check the cause is not something else like Crohn's disease, colitis or celiac disease (caused by a gluten intolerance).

People with IBS may need to avoid what are sometimes called fodmap foods. It stands for Fermentable Oligosaccharides, Disaccharides, Monosaccharides and Polyols. Snappy. They're basically various types of carbohydrate that are poorly absorbed by the body. Common offenders include onion, garlic, wheat and animal milks. If you think you might be affected, get some advice from a doctor or nutritionist.

Time can take its toll on our guts, especially if we've taken lots of antibiotics. Eating more slowly will help.

## Should I take probiotic supplements?

Probably not without guidance from a health professional. Theoretically, since we already have probiotics in our gut, supplements should be fine. But there have been question marks over whether probiotic supplements actually reach the gut alive. More recently, some research has suggested unwelcome side effects, especially in people with weakened immune systems.

## Soup up your vegetables

We are constantly being told that some berry or vegetable is a new superfood. I'd say forget superfoods and get into the souper-food. Soup can be a really easy and tasty way to eat better: a particularly handy trick for eating a good variety of vegetables.

A soup starter is less common in the UK than it was. Not so in China, where it's still the popular choice. It's great for portion control. Instead of wolfing down your main because you're starving, you'll eat more slowly and probably less.

Soup can also be a main course. A lot of us eat three times a day: breakfast, one big meal and one smaller one. The smaller meal is often a sandwich or something else that's a little easier to prepare (or buy at work). As the main part of this second meal, soup is ideal. It's not unusual in France, for example, to have soup in the evening if you've had your main meal at lunch.

You can make a big soup and then eat it over several days. Fresh, frozen or tinned vegetables – whatever you fancy, they'll all do. Hack all the fresh veg up small (carrots are a good one to include). In your saucepan, fry chopped onion in a little oil or butter. Add a bit of garlic if you like (it doesn't have to be fresh, buy paste). Add boiling water from the kettle and chuck in all the fresh veg. A little salt and pepper. Some herbs. Let the fresh stuff cook a little then add any frozen and then any tinned veg (a tin of tomatoes is a good choice). Let it all cook through nicely. Use a blender to whizz it all up, as the TV chefs say, and add some milk. Soya or almond are good as they're creamier.

Fancy croutons? Just lob in some cubes of stale bread, no frying or toasting needed. Less waste.

A souper-food that's souper easy and souper cheap. Sorry.

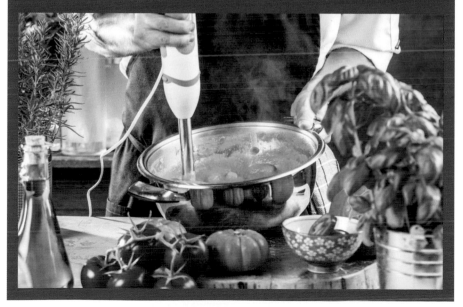

# Diabetes: fact from fiction

It seems everyone is talking about diabetes today. Should men be concerned? The answer is yes, but let's get the facts straight.

## How serious can it be? Steve Redgrave has diabetes and he's won five Olympic gold medals

Today, most of us know someone with diabetes and can even name at least one famous athlete with the condition. But this can give the impression that it is not very serious.

To be clear, undiagnosed, untreated diabetes can be very dangerous. It can kill. It doubles the risk of stroke and heart disease. It doubles the risk of depression. It increases the risk of erection problems and dementia. It also causes sight loss, kidney disease, kidney failure and nerve damage. Every week, more than 150 amputations are carried out because of diabetes, usually of toes, feet and legs, and this number is increasing.

But none of this is inevitable. Having diabetes doesn't mean you'll automatically go blind or have to give up your driving licence or never be able to travel or ever eat sugar or fruit again – all of these are common myths about diabetes. The truth is that diabetes, properly managed, does

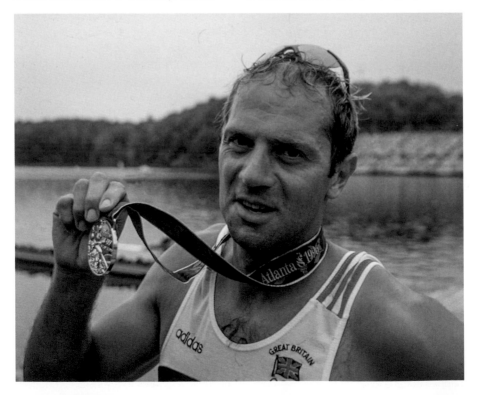

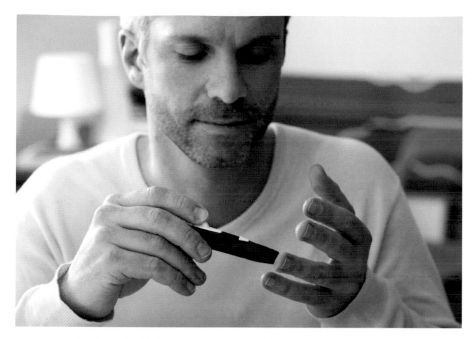

not stop you leading a full life. Many, many people do. Some of them pursue sporting or other high-profile careers. This doesn't prove that diabetes isn't serious. It proves that, if you take it seriously, you can live with diabetes. And live well.

Better to avoid it in the first place though, if you can.

## So what is diabetes?

Diabetes is a condition that causes your blood sugar level to become too high. This can damage blood supply to vital organs and lead to a variety of health problems.

## I'm none the wiser...

Our bodies convert food into energy. The main source of this energy is a sugar – glucose – which is created when food is digested. Glucose enters the bloodstream, where we call it blood sugar, and fuels the body's cells. But this process doesn't happen automatically.

The body uses the hormone insulin to allow glucose into the cells. Insulin is created in the pancreas, an organ that sits behind the stomach. The pancreas senses how much glucose has entered your blood and releases the right amount of insulin. This process doesn't work properly if you have diabetes.

## Aren't there two types of diabetes?

Yes. If your pancreas can't make any insulin at all, this is called type 1 diabetes. People with type 1 diabetes need to take replacement insulin.

Type 1 diabetes is usually diagnosed in children, but not exclusively. In fact, it is estimated about a quarter of new type 1 cases are in adults, sometimes adults in their eighties.

If your pancreas produces some, but not enough, insulin, or if your body's cells are unable to react to the insulin produced, it is called type 2 diabetes. Usually, people with type 2 are diagnosed as adults. They may be able to improve blood sugar control with diet and sometimes even put the diabetes into remission.

Most people with diabetes – 90% – have type 2 diabetes. About 8% have type 1 diabetes and 2% have rarer types.

## What's the risk?

Increasing. The number of people diagnosed with diabetes has more than doubled in 20 years. This is mainly type 2 diabetes, because we are getting heavier and being overweight is the major risk factor for type 2. However, type 1 is also currently increasing at a rate of about 2–5% per year worldwide.

One man in ten now has diabetes. Diabetes UK reckon that 12.3 million people are at increased risk of type 2 diabetes in the UK. Men are at greater risk: more UK men (68%) are overweight or obese than women (59%).

## But am I at risk?

You are at higher risk if you:

- Are aged over 40 (or 25 for south Asian people)
- Have a close relative with diabetes – such as a parent, brother or sister
- Are of south Asian, Chinese, African-Caribbean or black African origin (even if you were born in the UK)
- Are overweight or obese (especially if you have a lot of fat round your middle)
- Have high blood pressure and/or high cholesterol
- Have a lifestyle that involves a lot of sitting down
- Smoke.

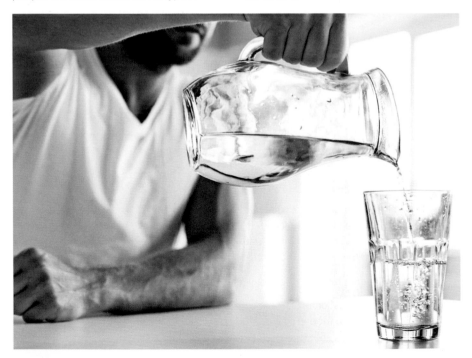

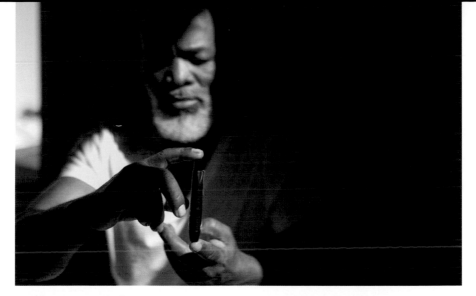

## What are the symptoms?

The symptoms of both types are much the same:

- Feeling unusually thirsty
- Peeing more than usual, especially at night
- Feeling unusually tired
- Frequent itching around the penis or even thrush
- Cuts or wounds healing more slowly
- Blurred vision
- Unexplained weight loss

Poor erections and reduced sex drive may also be warning signs for diabetes.

## Is diabetes my fault?

No. You can't do anything about type 1 diabetes and while it's true that you can reduce your risk of type 2 diabetes, it's not your fault if you do develop it. Indeed, there is evidence that our risk of type 2 diabetes may be traced back to the genetic variants introduced when modern humans interbred with Neanderthals 40,000–80,000 years ago – so definitely not your fault.

If you think you may have diabetes, see your GP.

---

**CASE STUDY**

# GEORGE: I'M PRE-DIABETIC

The GP told me I was pre-diabetic at a routine check-up. I felt tired. My face felt bloated. My skin was red and itchy. I just thought I was run down – I didn't put it down to what I was eating.

Now I eat more fruit and veg. And I drink water. I used to just drink Lucozade.

I started reading the food labels but they're very confusing when it comes to sugar. If you look at apple juice, it has loads of sugar but is it artificial or natural? It's better to eat an apple than drink an apple juice.

*By keeping an eye on diet and exercise, George has avoided developing diabetes.*

# Drink talking

Alcohol is probably the most popular drug in the world. Like any drug, if you're going to take it, you need to know how it works.

At its best, alcohol can be part of the fun of being with people. At its worst, it can kill. Second only to tobacco as a killer, alcohol is responsible for five times more deaths worldwide than all the illegal drugs put together. Part of knowing how it works is knowing that anyone at any time could develop a problem with alcohol, including you.

The trouble is that we don't quite understand alcohol, especially when we're drinking it. One drink may well help you to relax at a party and have more fun, but that doesn't mean that you'll have ten times as much fun if you have ten drinks. Alcohol encourages you to forget this fact.

In the UK, the chief medical officers remind us that there is no absolutely safe level of drinking. They advise no more than 14 units a week, including some alcohol-free days. They also advise against binge-drinking – defined, for men, as over eight units in a session.

## What is a unit?

A unit is 10 millilitres (ml) of alcohol, which is about two teaspoonfuls.

The standard drinks sold in bars may all

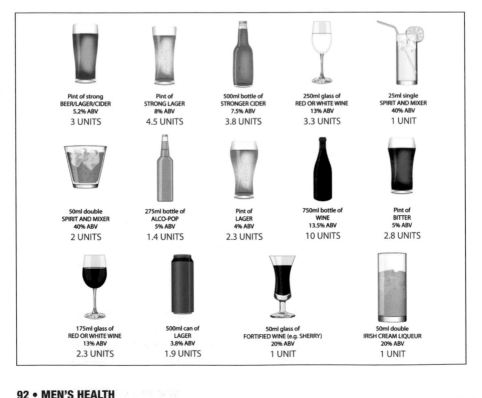

| | | | | |
|---|---|---|---|---|
| Pint of strong BEER/LAGER/CIDER 5.2% ABV **3 UNITS** | Pint of STRONG LAGER 8% ABV **4.5 UNITS** | 500ml bottle of STRONGER CIDER 7.5% ABV **3.8 UNITS** | 250ml glass of RED OR WHITE WINE 13% ABV **3.3 UNITS** | 25ml single SPIRIT AND MIXER 40% ABV **1 UNIT** |
| 50ml double SPIRIT AND MIXER 40% ABV **2 UNITS** | 275ml bottle of ALCO-POP 5% ABV **1.4 UNITS** | Pint of LAGER 4% ABV **2.3 UNITS** | 750ml bottle of WINE 13.5% ABV **10 UNITS** | Pint of BITTER 5% ABV **2.8 UNITS** |
| 175ml glass of RED OR WHITE WINE 13% ABV **2.3 UNITS** | 500ml can of LAGER 3.8% ABV **1.9 UNITS** | 50ml glass of FORTIFIED WINE (e.g. SHERRY) 20% ABV **1 UNIT** | 50ml double IRISH CREAM LIQUEUR 20% ABV **1 UNIT** | |

be different sizes but, in theory, they have about one unit of alcohol in them. One unit = one 30ml glass of spirit (a single measure) = one 100ml glass of wine = half a pint of ordinary 3.5% beer.

It's not a great guide, though. Many beers are far stronger. Watch out for glass sizes too. Some large wine glasses hold a third of a bottle. And then there are cocktails....

Information on units of alcohol is not user-friendly. Most bottles and tins carry some information from which you can – if you have a degree in advanced mathematics – work out how much alcohol you are actually drinking.

For example, say you have a 33cl (centilitre) can of beer, which contains 6% alcohol. This 33cl equals 330ml (millilitre), so you multiply 330 by 0.06. This means that there is 19.8ml of alcohol in the can, which is about two units. Confused? (Need a drink?)

## What does the body do with alcohol?

Like anything you eat or drink, booze goes down your throat and into your stomach. However, while most food stays there to be broken down by the stomach, alcohol doesn't. Alcohol is all over you like a rash.

Thirty seconds after your first sip it reaches the brain. Here it slows down the messages your brain sends to the rest of your body. You feel more relaxed but already it means that there are some things you will find more difficult to do, such as driving, riding a bike, operating machinery or answering questions in the pub quiz.

Full stomach or empty stomach, you'll still be affected. You may notice the alcohol more quickly if you drink on an empty stomach, while a full stomach may mean that the alcohol goes into the blood more

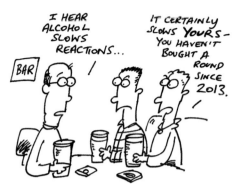

I HEAR ALCOHOL SLOWS REACTIONS...

IT CERTAINLY SLOWS YOURS – YOU HAVEN'T BOUGHT A ROUND SINCE 2013.

BAR

slowly, but in the end it's the same story. You get drunk.

The alcohol is finally processed in the liver. It takes the liver about an hour to break down one unit of alcohol fully. That means that after an hour, the unit will no longer affect you – unless, of course, you've had another drink.

## The liver doesn't like alcohol much, right?

It's not wild about it, no. Even after just a few drinks, your liver can feel tender and painful the next day.

Two facts: deaths from liver disease have increased by 400% since the 1970s and the main cause of liver disease, by far, is alcohol. If you have liver disease, you need to stop drinking because over time liver disease becomes irreversible.

### Quick Win

*Find a soft drink*
*Find a soft drink you like (preferably low sugar) and order it in the pub. Mine is lime cordial and soda. Making your first drink a soft one (or water) will help cut alcohol consumption. It'll quench your thirst and rehydrate you too. Zero-alcohol wines and beers taste better than they did too.*

## How does alcohol affect other parts of the body?

Alcohol slows the brain down sooner and for longer than we think. It begins after a unit or less and is still there the next day. A brain affected by alcohol both makes more mistakes and becomes less likely to notice them.

Too much alcohol can cause heart disease and high blood pressure, stomach problems such as ulcers and cancers of the throat, mouth and tongue.

Alcohol is fattening (a pint of beer contains about 185 calories – 30 more than a 28g packet of crisps) and also makes you feel hungry. Put the two together and what have you got? The beer belly or, to put it another way, fat in the most dangerous place for heart disease.

Last but not least, there's sex. Alcohol increases desire but reduces performance. Because of the effect of alcohol on the brain – where erections begin – and on blood flow into the penis, it can make erections poorer. In practice, while one drink might help you to get an erection, several won't and with heavy, long-term drinking, erectile dysfunction can become regular. Longer term, frequent heavy boozing can shrink your testicles and lower sperm count.

Perhaps this is just nature's way of preventing us from doing something we might regret in the morning. (Studies suggest 'beer goggles' really do exist.)

## What about mental health?

Drink can make you depressed. Depression can make you drink. A vicious circle. Alcohol is frequently involved in crime, domestic violence and suicide.

## What causes a hangover?

Alcohol makes you pee, reducing the amount of water in your brain and body, causing headaches. It disrupts your sleep and, of course, your stomach and liver. Add these up and you have that familiar morning-after feeling. Drinking water before going to bed may help make the hangover less unpleasant.

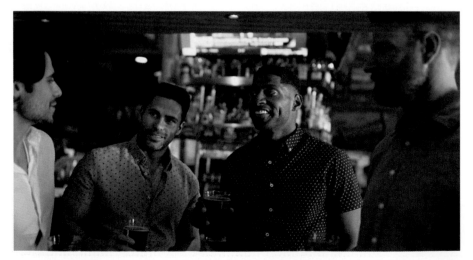

We're all differently affected by alcohol. Your size and metabolism make a difference. So does the time of day and the reason why you're choosing to have a drink in the first place. To repeat, anyone can develop a problem with alcohol. An early warning sign that you might be at risk is getting drunk very easily and/or having memory blackouts when you drink and can't remember what happened.

It's no more your fault that you have no control over alcohol than it is that you have brown eyes. The tough thing is admitting it. It's perhaps the toughest call you'll ever have to make, but if you don't, alcohol may well kill you.

Some people with alcohol problems are masters at hiding it from both other people and themselves. Alcoholism is a disease that tells you that you don't have it. If you're worried about yourself, that alone should be a warning to cut down. If you can't cut down, you have to stop. Check out the section on addiction on page 130–1.

The risk of alcohol is increased if you mix it with other drugs – legal or illegal. If you're on medication, check how much you can drink with your GP.

## Twelve tips for cutting down

1  Keep a drink diary – just seeing it in black and white can help.
2  Always know how much you've drunk. An app may help. Check labels to know exactly how much alcohol you're consuming.
3  Team up with your partner or mates to support each other.
4  Don't get into big rounds or drinking schools.
5  Have a soft drink or water every so often. Perhaps make your first drink a soft one.
6  Give up drink for a week, a month, the summer or until Spurs next reach the Champions League final.
7  Say 'no' from time to time.
8  Avoid mixing drinks.
9  Set clear goals. Don't be vague. Set a specific maximum for specific days or events. Limit yourself to a certain amount of money.
10 Know your motivations. Make a list of the reasons you want to cut down: improved health, more energy, better sex, better relationships, saving money, being fitter etc. And keep them close.
11 Know your triggers. People, places, times. If, for example, you always have one after work, give yourself a distraction (a walk, exercise, computer game, whatever) to break the association. Miss the company? Go for a coffee instead.
12 Try some nudges at home. Have less drink (or even no drink) indoors. If you feel the urge to finish a bottle, buy a smaller bottle (or a screw top). Use an alcohol measure so you don't always pour yourself 'a large one'. Try a 'no beer in the fridge' rule, which means you have to choose to have one rather than just grabbing one because it's there.

If you can't do these things, then you don't need to cut down, you need to stop.

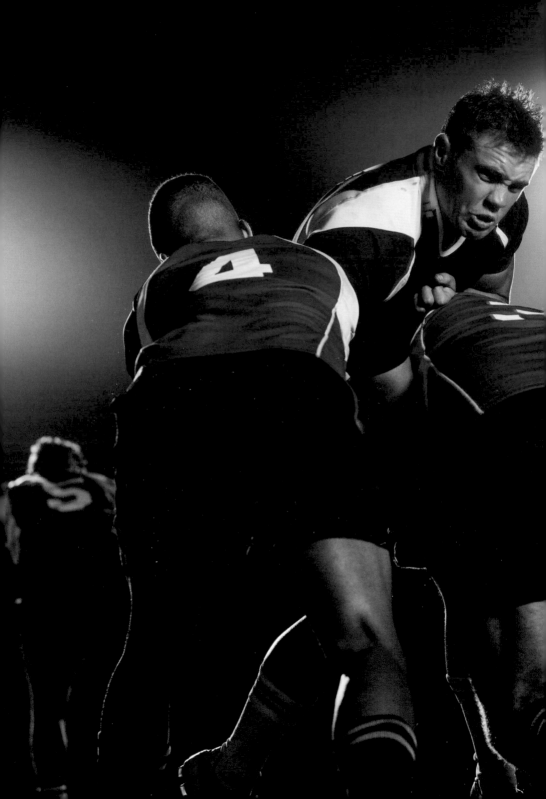

# Chapter 5

# How to handle your tackle

Everything that is good for your heart is also good for your tackle and your erections.

Why? Because an erection is the result of blood flooding into the penis. If the blood is not flowing properly, then the erection won't happen properly. The blood pressure inside an erect penis is very high – 700 mmHg or more (140 mmHg is generally considered 'high' blood pressure outside of the penis). It takes a good, efficiently pumping heart to provide this.

What this means is that any problems getting an erection could be an early sign of heart disease: one of a number of reasons why you need to take erectile dysfunction (ED) seriously.

Many of the examples given in this section are drawn from heterosexual relationships but the basic information applies to all men regardless of partner preference.

# What happens when you ejaculate?

Sperm are manufactured in the testicles and pass along the epididymis, where the mature sperm hang out. The epididymis is a microscopically narrow tube, 6 metres long, folded into a space of just 5 centimetres – an engineering masterpiece.

Just before orgasm, the sperm travel along two narrow tubes of muscle called the vas deferens. These meet with the seminal vesicles, which are behind the bladder and just above the prostate gland. The seminal vesicles and the prostate add their own secretions to the semen. These alkaline fluids protect the sperm from the acid in the vagina. At orgasm, the semen is propelled from two ejaculatory ducts along the urethra, which runs the length of the penis, and out of the urethral opening.

The average ejaculation contains 200–300 million sperm, but it only takes one to fertilise the egg. (Just as well, because only about 40 of them will get anywhere near the end of the race.)

Sperm are tadpole-shaped and about 0.05mm long. From puberty onwards, at least 1,000 sperm are manufactured each minute in the testicles. They take

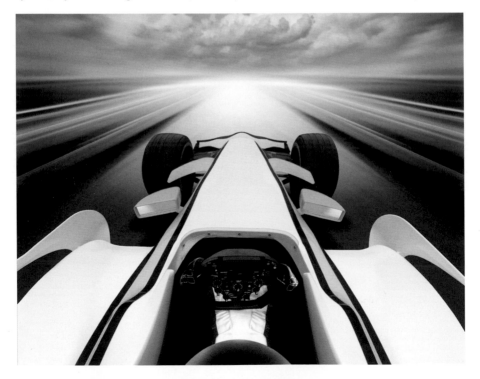

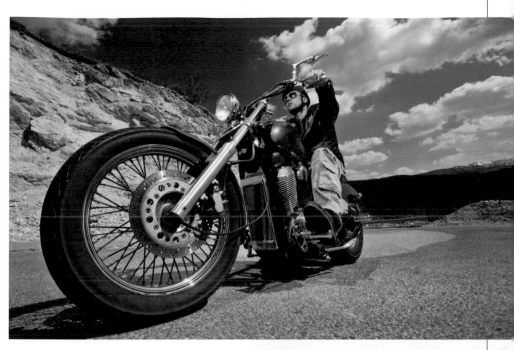

about two and a half months to mature
and spend the last couple of weeks in
the epididymis.

Sperm swim at about 15cm (6in) a
second but at the point of ejaculation they
are propelled a lot faster – about 45kph
(28mph) – along with the rest of the
seminal fluid. Two minutes after entering
the female, they're at the cervix and five
minutes later they're at the fallopian tubes.

During the most fertile part of the
female menstrual cycle (period), the
sperms' journey is much easier because at
this time there is plenty of fertile mucus
around for the sperm to live off. They can
survive like this for – take a deep breath,
non-condom users – a week. The
woman's most fertile period is when the
egg is released – usually between the 12th
and 18th day of the cycle. If you and your
partner are trying for a baby, this is when
you'll be at it like Olympic athletes.

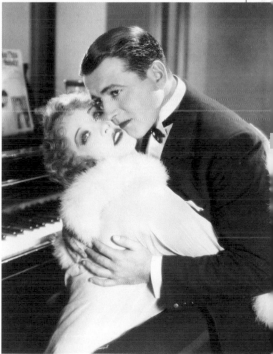

# Is my penis too small?

Penises come in all shapes and sizes, with bumps and bends and visible veins, the lot. Genuine problems that might actually stop you peeing or enjoying sex are rare and usually picked up when you're very young, so if you got through the nappy stage then you're probably good to go.

Most penises, when they're erect, are about the same length (between about five and a half and six and a quarter inches long). However, the exact size varies a lot, according to who measures it. In surveys when a doctor measures penis size, it drops compared with surveys in which the owner measures it. One of the reasons why some men may think they have small dicks is because the famous Kinsey report, which first talked about penis size, suggested the average was over six inches. The problem? It relied on self-reporting from the men interviewed.

If you're worried about your penis size, have a proper look at it. When you look at your penis normally, you're looking down on it. It's like looking down on someone from the top of a building. Even basketball players look small when you look down on them from above.

Hold a mirror at the side and have a proper look. That's more the sort of view you get of another man's penis in the public lavatory. Honestly, very, very few men are over- or under-endowed to the point that they cannot enjoy great sex. Think about it – the vagina

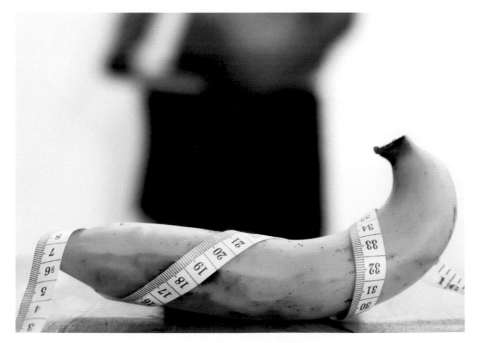

can be big enough to let a baby out or small enough to hold a tampon, which means it can cope with any size without loss of performance.

Ageing, obesity and some prostate operations may make the penis a little smaller. But nothing to stop you enjoying it.

Operations to enlarge the penis tend only to make it look bigger when limp and not when erect, and are – like any other surgery – potentially dangerous. You only have one penis. Although livers, kidneys and hearts can all be replaced if necessary, the penis cannot. Don't.

## Why is my erect penis bent?

Every penis is a bit bent, and a slight bend upward is not just normal but desirable. However, if your penis is bent to the left or right so much that it is difficult or even painful to enter your partner during sex, this could be a condition called Peyronie's disease (not an Italian beer). If the 'bend' is severe, surgery can improve matters. Men aged 50 to 60 are most at risk, although Peyronie's can occur at any age.

## Should I wash my knob?

Assuming you shower or bath regularly, no special cleaning is required.

Keep your penis clean, including under the foreskin. It is naturally smelly at best, and after a day or so that nasty white stuff – smegma – starts to bloom. This can lead to a swollen glans (helmet), or balanitis (literally, 'inflammation of the acorn'). Washing with plain soap and a couple of handfuls of salt in the bath should sort balanitis out. If not, see your GP. Balanitis may also be caused by perfumes in soaps and gels or sex with a

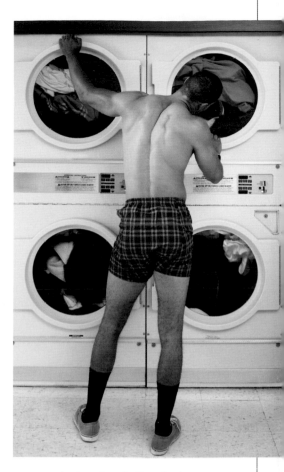

woman who has thrush. Poor hygiene can increase the risk of cancer of the penis, although this is rare.

Look after the groin area too. 'Jock itch', which is caused by the same tinea fungus as athlete's foot, thrives in warm, moist conditions – a good description of the average man's pants at the end of a busy day. Wash with unperfumed soaps, dry thoroughly and – superheroes take note – avoid tight nylon underpants. See your doctor if the problem persists.

Unless you're trying to have a baby, wear a condom to protect against STDs (sexually transmitted diseases) and HIV.

# Why can't I get an erection?

Not getting an erection when you want one is usually called ED (erectile dysfunction). You may still hear it called impotence.

The official estimate is that ED affects about one in ten men at any one time, but surveys vary and some have put it far higher. The general rule of thumb is that the risk increases with age, with about 40% of men affected at age 40 and about 70% at age 70. That doesn't mean that ED is the inevitable result of ageing. It simply reflects the fact that older men are more likely than younger ones to have the

conditions that can cause ED. However, there is evidence that far more young people are now experiencing ED. Of men seeking treatment for the condition, as many as one in four are under 40. When younger men are affected, the condition may also be more severe.

ED is one of the things about being a flesh-and-blood human rather than a robot. If it happens occasionally, don't

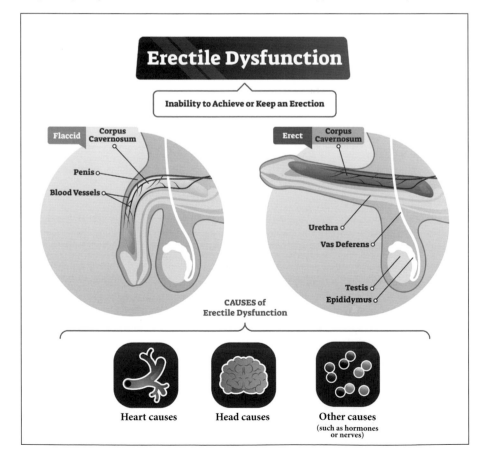

**Erectile Dysfunction**

Inability to Achieve or Keep an Erection

Flaccid — Corpus Cavernosum

Penis

Blood Vessels

Erect — Corpus Cavernosum

Urethra

Vas Deferens

Testis

Epididymus

CAUSES of Erectile Dysfunction

Heart causes

Head causes

Other causes (such as hormones or nerves)

worry about it, but if it keeps happening see a doctor. Why? Because ED can be an early warning of some serious health problems including:

- Heart disease
- Narrow arteries
- High blood pressure
- Diabetes
- Peyronie's disease
- Multiple sclerosis
- Heavy drinking or smoking
- Drugs – either the side effects of prescribed drugs (e.g. some anti-depressants and drugs for high blood pressure) or the abuse of non-prescribed drugs.

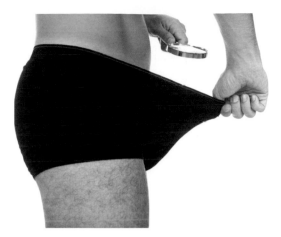

Research suggests that many men with ED don't seek help because they don't think it can be treated. This is not true. There are many causes of ED, both physical and psychological, but it can nearly always be treated. There is usually some physical cause; it is purely psychological in only about 25% of cases. Whatever the cause, worrying about sexual performance can make it worse. This is because anxiety contracts the muscles, preventing blood from entering the penis.

If you get erections at night or when masturbating but have problems with your partner, it's almost certainly not a physical problem so just relax. The chances are you'll live to 80, so there's plenty of time.

As usual, smoking is a no-no. Nicotine interferes with the flow of blood to the penis, making an erection less likely. Smokers are one and a half to three times more likely to have ED than non-smokers. Engrave it on your lighter.

Being overweight is a factor for high blood pressure and diabetes, meaning it's also a factor for ED. More exercise and less alcohol might help too.

ED can be treated using drugs that your doctor can prescribe or which can be bought over the counter in the pharmacy. You may be tempted to buy these off the internet, but you should only do so if you already have a doctor's prescription. Sites that will sell you drugs without a prescription could, frankly, be selling you anything, including fakes made with blue paint and pesticides. Also, if you don't see a doctor, the underlying cause – which may be far more serious than a bit of brewer's droop – won't be sorted out.

Some say pelvic floor exercises (or Kegels) may help. Clench and release the muscles you use to stop yourself peeing in mid-flow. Feels weird, though.

If you have the opposite problem, an erection all the time, this could be priapism – a painful condition that requires prompt treatment to avoid the risk of ED in the future and permanent damage to the penis. As a guide, any man whose erection continues for four hours or more should see a doctor. (Check out the Robert De Niro movie, *Young Fockers*, for further information.)

## What about testosterone?

Low testosterone levels are seldom the
cause of ED.

Increasing testosterone levels is more
likely to increase sex drive than improve
ED. Although a low testosterone level may
reduce your desire to go out and seek sex,
it shouldn't affect erections when sex is in
front of you. In other words, even if you
have low testosterone levels, seeing
something you find sexually exciting should
prompt an erection.

## If testosterone has nothing to do with erections, what is it for?

Testosterone is the most important of
the male hormones. It's made mostly in
the testicles but also in the adrenal
glands. (The ovaries and adrenal glands
produce it in lower levels in women.) In
men, it is responsible for muscle, bone
and sexual development, as well as sex
drive. At puberty, it makes the voice
drop and the penis, testicles, and facial
and pubic hair grow.

Women's hormones have been at the
forefront of health for decades now. Only
recently have the hormonal fluctuations
that men experience attracted much
interest. But the fact is that male mood,
behaviour and, indeed, health are heavily
influenced by our hormones, especially
testosterone. Testosterone levels fluctuate
according to circumstances. They can rise
before and, if successful, after conflict.
They can fall after marriage or the birth of
a child.

Overall, testosterone levels fall slightly
with age. Some men – particularly those
with high levels to begin with – can
effectively have half as much testosterone
in their blood at 80 as at 20. It may lead to
loss of muscle tone and bone strength,

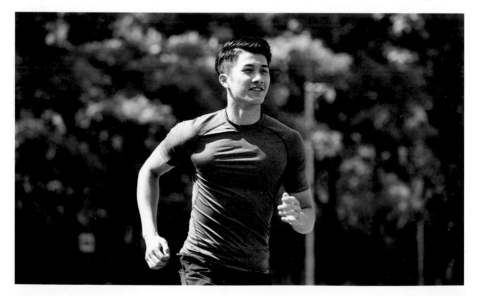

and increased weight and risk of heart disease and diabetes. Moreover, the well-known Massachusetts Male Aging Study suggests there may be a generational decrease in testosterone levels – in other words, men of a certain age now have lower testosterone levels than men of the same age in the past.

Whether reduced testosterone is the cause of the sluggishness, loss of libido and depression that some middle-aged men experience is debatable. It may be the result of low mood rather than the cause of it. (Depressed men often have low levels of testosterone and high levels of cortisol, the hormone released in response to stress.)

Testosterone replacement therapy (TRT) is available and used to treat some cases of low testosterone. But, while trials continue, many doctors are sceptical about its wider use and endocrinologists (the doctors who deal with hormones) are concerned about over-diagnosis of low testosterone in men, especially as there are some groups in which TRT is not advised. There are major side effects to taking testosterone artificially. It can affect the heart, prostate and even your fertility. This is because when your brain notices your testosterone is high, it tells your testicles to stop making it. The trouble is that when they stop making testosterone, they also stop producing sperm. Result: infertility. It happens so often some have suggested testosterone as a contraceptive. Yes, really.

## Can you boost testosterone levels naturally?

Yes. By taking more exercise, having more sex, making sure you get your essential fatty acids and getting a good night's

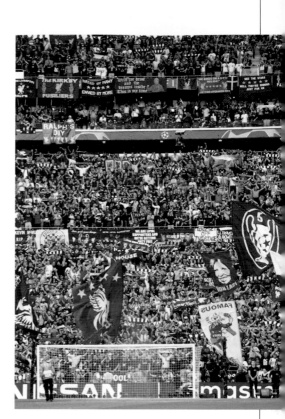

sleep. Also, fat reduces the amount of testosterone available to the body, so losing weight and cutting down on fatty foods and beer may help.

Eat more seeds (particularly pine nuts, pumpkin and sunflower seeds), shellfish (including shrimp and oysters), beans, yoghurt and lean meat. These are high in zinc, which is the mineral that is essential for testosterone production. Oats, honey, broccoli, spinach, cauliflower, radishes, turnips, cabbage and Brussels sprouts can help too, as can ginseng, the South American herb Muira Puama, and even stinging nettles (better in a tea than raw!)

A good natural boost could be to support a better football team. Testosterone levels rise in supporters of winning teams and decline in supporters of losing teams.

# Are sperm counts falling?

They appear to be. Research suggests that during the past 50 years or so, the number of sperm in the average Western male's semen has halved.

What doctors call a 'normal' sperm level today is just a third of the 'normal' level in the 1940s. The rapid decline suggests the problem is linked to lifestyle and the environment, with the finger being pointed at plastics containing 'endocrine disruptors'.

When it comes to infertility, the man will be part of the problem in around half of cases, with low sperm count (called oligospermia) the most frequent reason. All of the following can reduce sperm count:

■ Anabolic steroids (very severely)
■ Anti-arthritis drugs
■ Alcohol
■ Cocaine
■ Chemotherapy
■ Frequent marijuana use
■ Low levels of minerals such as zinc
■ Low levels of vitamins, particularly vitamin C
■ Smoking (reduces the sperm's life expectancy and sense of direction)
■ Some other prescription drugs (this includes ED drugs like Viagra, which is a good argument against 'recreational' use of these drugs by men who might want to start families)
■ Stress
■ A vasectomy, which may not be as reversible as is sometimes believed.

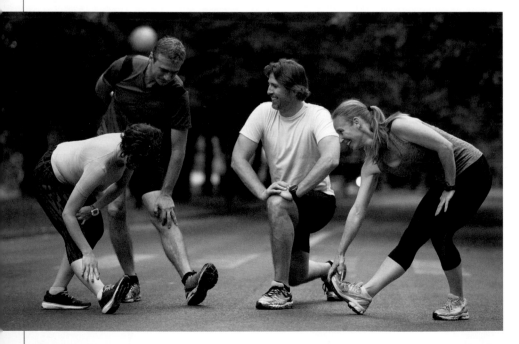

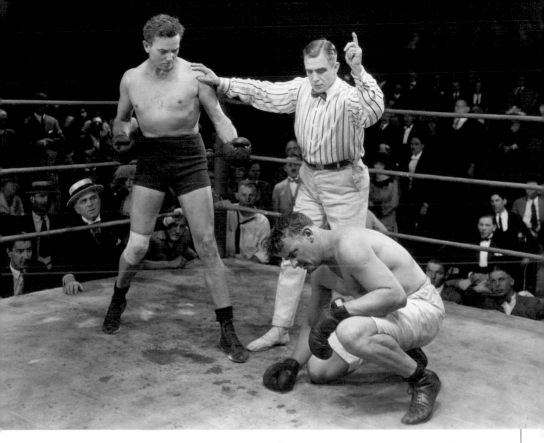

Some like it hot but not sperm. They thrive at about three degrees below body temperature. This is why your testicles are outside the body. It also means baggy trousers and boxers are best for baby making.It's not clear whether the increase in testicular cancer is linked to falling sperm counts. Although still rare, cases of testicular cancer have more than doubled in the same time that sperm counts have halved.

Although the number of people getting testicular cancer is up, deaths are down. In fact, since the early 1970s, deaths from testicular cancer have gone down by 83% in UK males. An undescended testicle when an infant is a risk factor for testicular cancer. This cancer is more common in white men than Asian or black men.

## Should I check my testicles for cancer?

The best way to monitor your own body for ill health is simply to be aware of it. Testicular cancer is rare and, if caught in time, nearly always treatable. Because of this, although it's still the most common cancer among men under 50, more men die of breast cancer than testicular cancer.

Rather than checking your testicles religiously and fretting over whether you're doing it properly, just be aware. When you examine your balls you will feel a lump on the top towards the back where the epididymis joins. This will be there every time, obviously. You're looking out for other lumps and/or heaviness. If you're concerned, see your GP.

# Let's talk about sex

Regular sex is good for you, provided it's safe. It reduces stress, boosts the immune system, enhances self-esteem, aids sleep, burns calories and improves intimacy with your partner. It can even reduce pain. The way to make it 100% safe is to use a condom.

As men, we don't always appreciate that good sex actually happens in the head. I say this not just because so much of our sex lives involve fantasy, but also because good sex comes from feeling comfortable in ourselves about our bodies and our sexuality.

Celebrate your sexuality. 'Safe sex doesn't mean no sex, it just means use your imagination' is how Billy Bragg put it in his hit single 'Sexuality'. Like the bard of Barking says, your sexuality is all yours. It's part of you. Don't be ashamed of what you like.

The mouth is an important sex organ too – being able to talk honestly about sex with your partner is as important as doing it. Tell each other what you like. Do what you like, so long as it's legal and between consenting adults.

I'm now going to talk about some issues that may not at first glance appear to have anything to do with your health. I mention them because, if you're affected by them, they can have major implications for your mental and physical health.

## Is masturbation bad for you?

No. It won't make you go blind, vote Monster Raving Looney or put you off your cornflakes. Most men masturbate and, despite what they might say, so do many women. It's perfectly normal. After all, our genitals are part of our bodies and pretty important to our relationships, so it would be surprising if we weren't just a little curious about them.

In fact, masturbation can be good for you. It will help you to understand your body, your sexuality and what turns you on

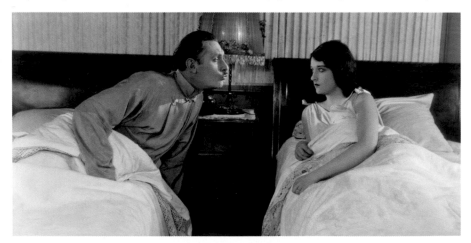

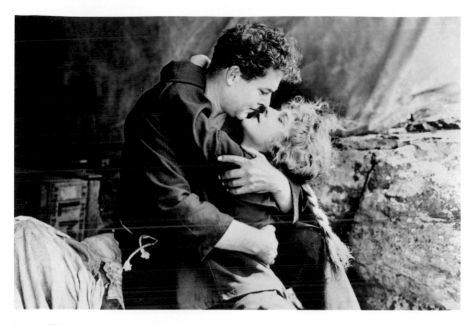

better. This may help you communicate with your partner more easily, enjoy sex more and avoid sex-related psychological problems. (Indeed, masturbating with your partner is a good way to show each other what you like.) Frequent orgasms also help to reduce the risk of prostate cancer, and masturbation itself also reduces the likelihood of phimosis – a tightness of the foreskin. Furthermore, although nobody has yet begun to promote masturbation as part of a calorie-controlled diet, it does definitely burn a few. Some men claim their wearable-tech thinks they're walking when they're actually otherwise engaged. How many calories? 50 plus maybe? The truth is nobody really knows because despite most science students being young males with traditional young male interests, no specific research has been done.

The need for sexual pleasure is a natural human need, the same as the need for food and drink, and when the urge strikes it is surely better to masturbate than exploit someone else who may not fancy it as much as you.

Having said all that, your penis is a delicate body part. Take care of it – don't stick it in anything other than your partner or stick anything else into it.

Anything that is enjoyable can become an addiction, and masturbation is no different. If it begins to interfere with the rest of your life and you're becoming more interested in it than in real sexual relationships with real people, then you need to be careful. Are you using it to cope with difficult feelings or problems? Perhaps it sometimes makes you feel crap about yourself afterwards. If you can't stop, you need to. Just as for other addictions, there are organisations for people who are addicted in this way, such as Sexaholics Anonymous.

## Is it OK to use pornography?

When you're a teenager, looking at porn is part of a normal curiosity, but using it when

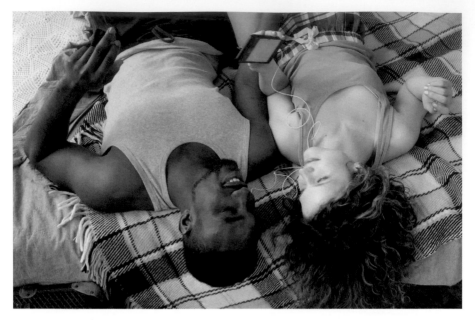

you're older depends more on your view of the politics of porn and its effects.

It is true that some women enjoy pornography aimed at heterosexual men, even including some of the women who appear, but – as with prostitution – this is the exception rather than the rule and there is widespread abuse of women in the porn industry. Pornography, by definition, exploits women by treating them as objects for sexual pleasure. Because you can't avoid that, regular use may affect your attitudes to women and spoil your relationships with them.

Be careful – you can get addicted to pornography too.

## What about prostitution?

Selling sex is legal but a lot of the things surrounding it are illegal, including selling it in the street, pimping or running a brothel.

Paying for sex is legal. But it is illegal to buy from anyone under 18 or from anyone who has been forced into it. You can be committing a crime even if you honestly didn't know they were being forced.

As with pornography, you can kid yourself as much as you like that, because it's legal, you're doing nothing wrong, but the fact of the matter is that although a few prostitutes may enjoy their work, many more are abused or do it unwillingly.

## What's the law?

Historically, the law in most countries has been uncomfortable and confused about sexuality but today it tries to look at the actors rather than the act.

There are few acts between consenting adults that are illegal, but all this changes if the people involved are relatives or if one of them is under the age of consent (16 in the UK).

There is help available for anyone who thinks about, or who acts outside the law.

The Lucy Faithfull Foundation run a project called Stop it Now (www.stopitnow. org.uk), which has a helpline for people seeking help with their own abusive behaviour or feelings (freephone 0808 1000 900). It also provides support for those who suspect someone they know presents a risk.

## What are the symptoms of a sexually transmitted infection?

Sexually transmitted infections (STIs), formerly known as VD (venereal disease), are very common and can affect you whether you're straight, gay or bisexual. You don't need to have lots of partners to be at risk – one brief encounter with a person with an STI may be enough. They can be transmitted through vaginal sex, oral sex, anal sex and, in some cases, through skin-to-skin contact. (HIV cannot be passed via skin-to-skin contact.)

As a rule, STIs can be cured or safely treated if they're caught early. If not, they can become more serious, possibly causing infertility or even death.

Some of the more common symptoms to look out for include:

- An unusual discharge from your penis
- Swollen testicles

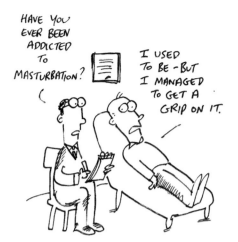

- Itching, rashes, lumps or soreness in the penis or tackle region
- Pain when peeing. (A short-term stinging sensation when peeing may be cystitis – drink plenty of water and it should improve.)

If you or your partner have any of these symptoms, or any other sexual health concerns, see a GP or a specialist sexual health clinic.

You can buy self-testing kits for some STIs in pharmacists, but use them with care. If you

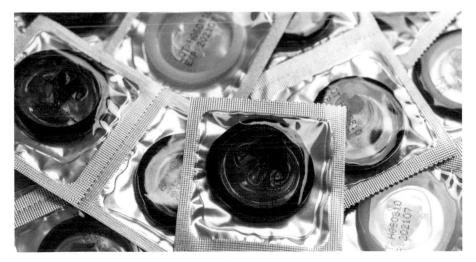

have one STI, you've possibly got another, so it still makes sense to see a doctor.

STIs are on the increase in the UK. The best way to avoid them is through safe sex. If you aren't safe and are concerned that you might have caught something, get yourself checked out, even if you don't have any symptoms. Some STIs such as chlamydia (about half of all new STI cases) and HIV often cause no symptoms at first.

## I know condoms are best but it just doesn't feel so good

It's not a case of one-size-fits-all. Condoms vary considerably in size, shape and thickness. Widely available condoms vary by over 20mm in length and by over 10mm in circumference. If you find one type is uncomfortable, shop around until you find another that suits you better.

On the plus side, some men say that wearing a condom makes sex last longer. That can't be a bad thing.

## Is blood at orgasm a symptom of an STI?

Blood in the semen can be very scary but is usually harmless. Very rarely it can be a sign of something more serious, so see a doctor if it happens more than once.

## What about blood when you pee?

Is it definitely blood? If you have not been drinking enough water your urine can begin to look brown. Certain foods, like beetroot, or certain drugs can also make your urine change colour.

If it is blood, it could be caused by an infection of the urinary tract or it could be the sign of something more serious such as a prostate problem. See your GP and try to take a urine sample.

A heavy workout can also cause the urine to look red, although it's not actually blood. If this keeps happening, see your doctor.

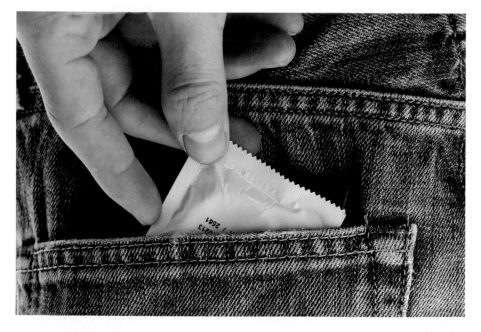

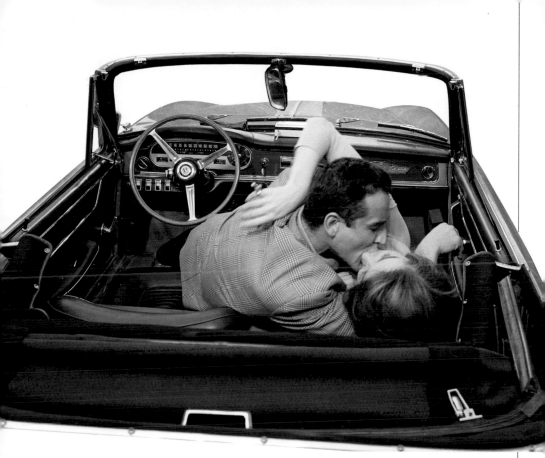

## I've got enough kids – should I have a vasectomy?

Vasectomies are less popular than they once were. About 12,000 are performed on the NHS every year, half the number carried out ten years ago. Partly it's men being less keen, partly it's NHS cuts.

The official line is that vasectomy is a routine procedure that is 99.8% effective for preventing pregnancy and after which the vast majority of men enjoy the same sex life as before. But I've spoken to a number of men who have had post-vasectomy pain and poor or no erections.

The NHS offers two types of vasectomy including a no scalpel option. In both types, the vas deferens (the two tubes that carry sperm from the testicles) are cut and then sealed or tied. It could be that the sperm, which has nowhere to go after this, builds up and causes swelling and pain.

The official line is changing. When I wrote an article about this in 2006, a year in which nearly 30,000 NHS vasectomies were carried out, the advice on the official NHS website said: 'There are no known long-term risks from a vasectomy.' It gives much more information now. If you're considering a vasectomy, I'd check out what other men say about it, as well as health professionals. You might ask your doctor if he's had one.

Vasectomies can be reversed but not generally on the NHS.

# The prostate: the sex organ where size matters

The prostate sits between the bladder and urethra (the tube through which you pee) and provides some of the fluids that make up the semen when you ejaculate. It contracts during orgasm, probably heightening the pleasure. It's also the one sex organ where size really does matter. In this case, small is beautiful.

About the size of a walnut in an adult, the prostate can, as a man gets older, grow to the size of an orange. This growth can make peeing difficult, reduce your interest in sex and cause erection problems.

## Why does it grow?

In the prostate gland, testosterone is broken down into the related hormone dihydrotestosterone, which appears to be involved in both baldness and the enlarged prostate. This doesn't mean that high or low levels of testosterone cause prostate cancer (or baldness, for that matter). It's more about the way your body reacts to a normal amount.

Most prostates grow. Usually the growth is not caused by cancer but in some cases it can become cancerous. By the age of 70, many men will have some degree of prostate cancer. The question is how aggressive it is.

Doctors will often follow a treatment they like to call 'watchful waiting', which basically means doing nothing but carrying out regular tests. It's very common in prostate growth. They're trying to work out whether the growth has become cancerous and how quickly the cells are multiplying.

## How dangerous is prostate cancer?

The number of prostate cancer cases in the UK has increased by over 40% since the 1990s. It is now the most common cancer in men and, after lung cancer, the second most common cause of cancer death. However, survival rates are also improving – they've tripled in the last 40 years or so.

Prostate cancer is still rare in men under 50. But generally, the younger you are, the more aggressive a cancer is likely to be. Recent research has suggested taller men might also be more likely to have aggressive cancers.

There's a strong family link. Your risk of prostate cancer is more than doubled if you have an affected brother or father, and it increases still further with the number of

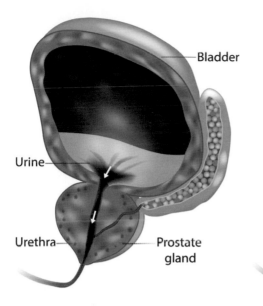

**Normal prostate**

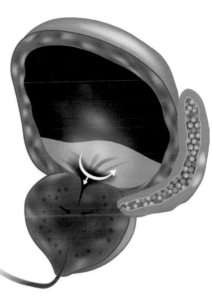

**Enlarged prostate gland**

male relatives you have with the disease. Prostate cancer is more common in black men than white and is least common in Asian men.

## What are the signs that my prostate might be growing?

Signs of an enlarged prostate include:

- **Weakness** – a weak, slower flow when you pee
- **Intermittency** – a flow that stops and starts
- **Hesitancy** – having to wait before you start to go
- **Frequency** – having to urinate more often than previously
- **Urgency** – finding it difficult to postpone urination
- **Nocturia** – having to get up at night to urinate.

If you have these symptoms and want to know whether they're likely to be prostate-related, ask yourself another question: is it easier and more satisfying peeing after having an orgasm? Some people with prostate problems find that it is, presumably as a result of the gland shrinking a little after it has added its vital fluid to your ejaculation.

## Is there a test for prostate cancer?

The reason men aren't called in for prostate cancer screening is that there isn't a simple, reliable test. The main test used is called the PSA. PSA stands for prostate specific antigen, a protein made in the prostate. Testing for this in the blood can be helpful, with a higher level suggesting that cancer is more likely. However, the test throws up a lot of false positives (high readings in men who don't, on further investigation, have cancer) and false negatives (low readings in men who do have cancer). For this reason, PSA as a single, one-off test is not reliable enough for screening. It is best used alongside other tests and examinations and used as a marker as part of 'watchful waiting'.

PSA is often used alongside the DRE (digital rectal examination). This may sound very high-tech but it's no more or less than the doctor's finger up your bottom to feel the prostate. If the prostate feels large or rough, further investigation is more likely. You're probably better off having a DRE from a urologist who specialises in these sorts of conditions than a GP who has probably done fewer. But research suggests the DRE is not always helpful either.

In the future, we hope that a more reliable test will allow for screening of men for prostate cancer. A variation of the ultrasound technique used to help diagnose breast cancer perhaps. Or, even better, a urine test which men may actually be able to do at home. Research continues on both these ideas.

Currently, urologists also use ultrasound, MRI and other scans to monitor the prostate. To be sure, a biopsy, where a piece of tissue from the prostate is examined under the microscope, is used.

## Sounds a bit hit and miss

It isn't. It just means diagnosis is a bit more complicated than it is for some other cancers. If you have any symptoms, see your GP. Whatever the cause, whether it is cancerous or not, doctors have a wide

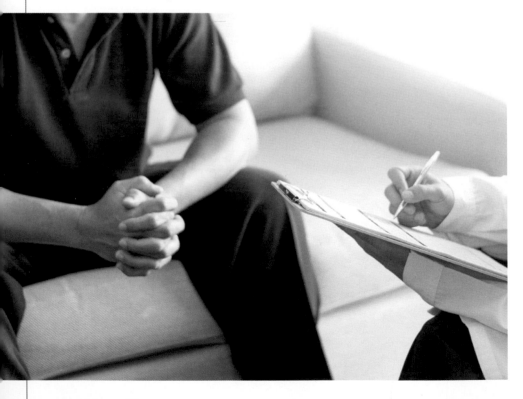

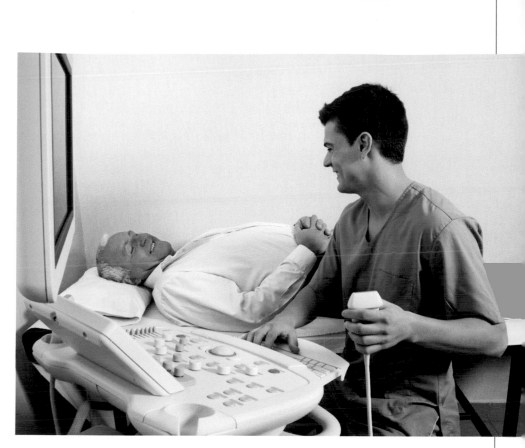

variety of treatments for enlarged prostates, from tablets to surgery and everything in between.

## What is good for the prostate?

A good, healthy diet with lots of antioxidants of the type we talked about on page 79 should help. You should also go easy on all the things you know you should go easy on, including alcohol. If you're taking any supplements or herbal remedies and need a PSA test, make sure your doctor knows what you're taking as they may interfere with the PSA result.

The big problem in prostate cancer research, more than in any other field, is that research tends to look at older men, but the key period that makes a difference could well come earlier in life, even in childhood. Having said that, one thing that does appear to help the prostate in the long term is frequent ejaculation.

An Australian study published in 2003 suggested men who had ejaculated more than five times per week in their twenties were one-third less likely to develop aggressive prostate cancer later. Subsequent research has drawn similar conclusions but there's a question about whether ejaculation can be solo or not. On one paper, frequent masturbation appeared to be a risk for prostate cancer in younger men but a protection against it in men over 50. The privilege of age. Whatever way you look at it, the prostate is a sex organ.

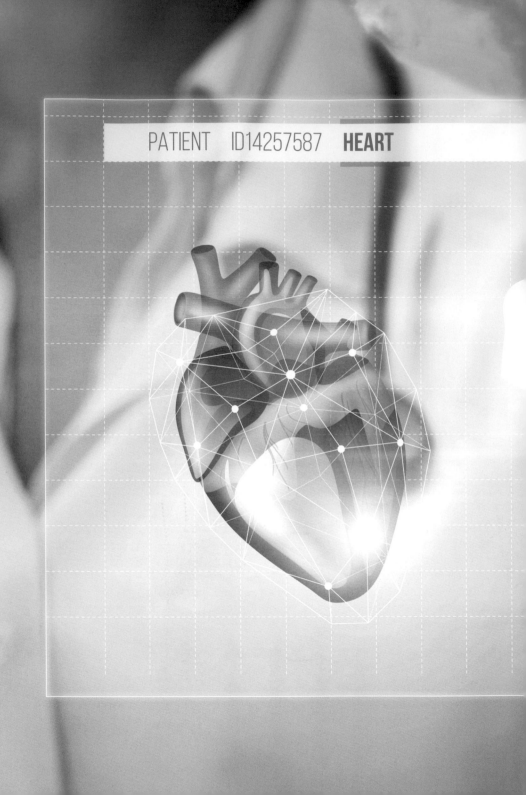

PATIENT   ID14257587   **HEART**

# Chapter 6

# Should I see someone?

If there's something you're not sure about, such as a pain, a lump or a cold, sore throat or stomach upset that won't clear up, the best bet is your general practitioner (GP). Only your GP can refer you to a specialist such as a hospital consultant or give you a prescription.

There are other useful health professionals at the GP surgery. The practice nurse, for example, can sort out holiday jabs and blood tests and explain how to use medicines or help with other routine matters, often without an appointment. Some surgeries also have physiotherapists, counsellors, blood pressure nurses and other specialists on site.

If you're not sure whether to go to the doctor or don't know which service to use, call 111. NHS 111 is open 24/7. They will send an ambulance if you need one.

There is now a useful NHS app for Apple and Android smartphones. It lets you check symptoms and find out what to do if you need help urgently. You can also link with most GP practices via the app.

# I don't have a GP

If you're not registered with a GP, pop into your local practice and ask to register as a patient. If they can't take you, they should point you to a nearby practice that can. You can search online for GP services at nhs.uk and find all practices in your area.

All GP surgeries should produce a leaflet explaining their services and most have a website too. Does your GP have extended opening hours? Over half of GP practices are now open in the evening or on Saturday to make it easier for working people to go.

When choosing a GP you might also want to think about: how easy it is to get to from home or work, parking and transport, how you book appointments, online services and how friendly the place feels.

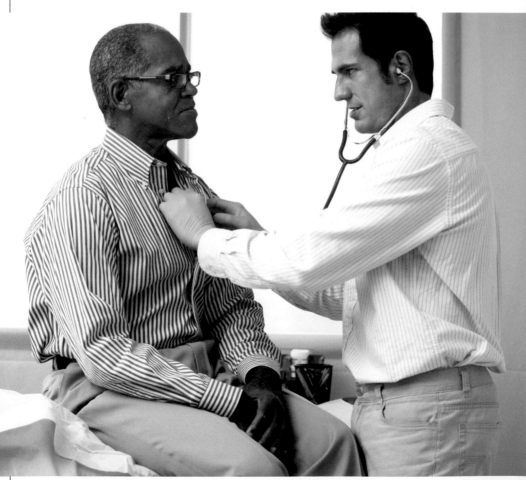

# Should I go to A&E?

A&E (accident and emergency) is also known as the emergency department or casualty. It is for emergencies and accidents. That's all.

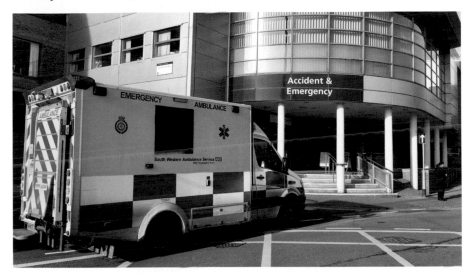

It deals with: bleeding that can't be stopped, severe burns, severe pain, broken bones, poisonings, overdoses, traumatic accidents and people who are unconscious or very confused.

If your problem is in one of these categories, get to A&E as soon as possible. You should get the help you need as promptly as you need it. Go for the wrong reason and you'll probably spend a long time hanging around. Umpteen men make this mistake every day.

Some people think that by ringing for an ambulance they will be seen as a priority. You won't. All new arrivals are assessed by a triage nurse who ensures that patients are seen in order of seriousness. Calling an ambulance when you don't need one may deny an ambulance to someone in a genuine life-or-death emergency.

TV programmes like *ER* can give the impression that A&E doctors are the best in their profession. This is not true. They are experts in accidents, but when it comes to, say, detecting a lump that could be cancerous, your GP is a much better starting point.

To deal with the overload at A&E, the NHS is pulling together a network of urgent treatment centres for when you need urgent medical attention but it's not a life-threatening situation. They're led by GPs and should be open at least 12 hours a day.

> You can find your nearest A& E and urgent treatment centre at nhs.uk. If you're not sure whether to go to the doctor or don't know which service to use, call 111. NHS 111 is open 24/7. They will send an ambulance if you need one.

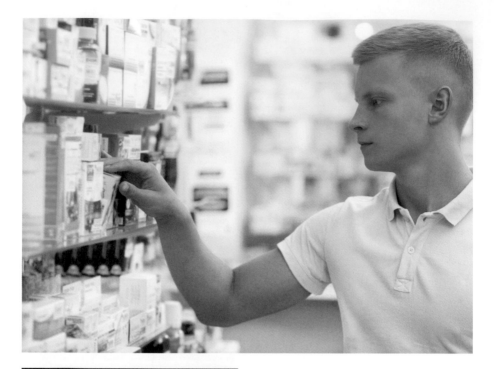

## NHS services you may not know about

- Sexual health clinics for sexually transmitted diseases and contraception (including emergency contraception)
- Specialist services around smoking, drugs and alcohol
- Mental health services – in some places you can just refer yourself to these without seeing your GP first
- Dental treatment is also cheaper on the NHS if you're lucky enough to find an NHS dentist
- In some cases, you might be entitled to free NHS eye tests.

There's information on all these services on nhs.uk.

## I don't really know how to talk to my doctor

It's not easy. Appointments are short and doctors are busy.

Try not to turn up with a list, but if you do, ask about your major concern first. Talk to your GP as you would to a friend, even when he or she doesn't seem particularly interested. For some doctors, the impersonal approach is a way of coping in a life-and-death profession.

Be honest. GPs have heard it all before. Don't be embarrassed, trivialise it or worry about wasting the doctor's time.

Make the most of the appointment. You might not have another one for a while. Make sure that you understand what your GP is saying. If not, ask for an explanation or more detail: 'What do you mean by a couple of tests?' Take a pen and a pad to take notes if you need to.

Be a patient patient. Doctors are doing their best under pressure but finding the right answer may take time. Don't expect instant solutions.

## My doc wants to do a 'procedure' – what's that?

A 'procedure' can be anything that is supposed to help diagnose your problem or treat it. Ask exactly what is being proposed. Blood tests won't do you any harm, and neither will the odd X-ray or scan. These are all over in seconds. If it's something longer like a colonoscopy, check you understand what's involved.

## Can't I just buy treatments myself?

Often you can. The high-street pharmacist is a health secret hidden in plain sight: a good source of quick medical advice. For many minor problems, it can be easier than going to the GP. Pharmacists can sell you over-the-counter (OTC) remedies for things like colds, sore throats, athlete's foot, dandruff or spots, and can tell you whether it's more serious than you think. No appointment needed and if you'd prefer to speak in private, just ask. It's normally no problem.

## It's affecting my health but it's not a health problem

Sometimes the help we need to feel better isn't medical. Work (or lack of it), housing, discrimination, emotional or physical domestic abuse, problems with children or other family members can all impact on our health. Citizens Advice is a good starting point to get help with these sorts of things.

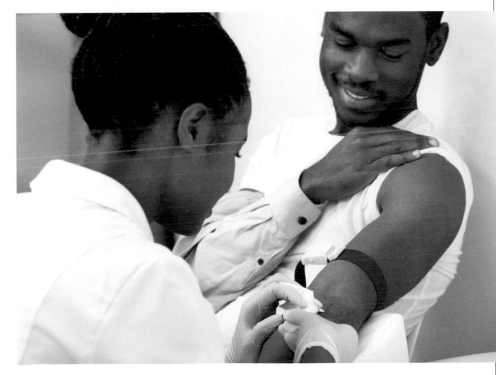

# What about the internet?

The web is great for research, but it's also full of junk. Googling 'men's health' will find you a billion results. The best places to start are the NHS website and the Men's Health Forum website. Both sites include plenty of links to other useful sources of info. As well as information and videos, many sites run by voluntary organisations now offer online services where you can chat with experts.

The NHS England Information Standard 'Health and care information you can trust' logo is a sign of quality. On overseas sites, look for the HONcode.

Be sceptical of social media, commercial sites or anyone using language like 'miracle cure'. Who runs the sites you're visiting? Many sites have an 'About us' section. If they don't, why not?

Look out for astroturfing (sites that look like they're grassroots, independent or charities but are actually a front for an organisation with a commercial or political point to make). Search engines may prioritise sites that are selling something, which is probably not what you want. Commercial sites also tend to be better at search engine optimisation than not-for-profits, patients' groups and academic institutions.

When researching online, be honest with yourself about what you do and don't know. We tend to think that social media

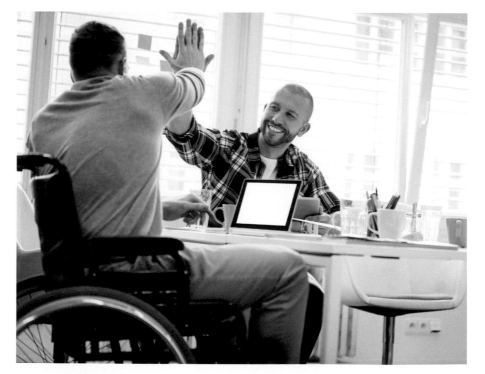

makes us an expert in everything. It doesn't. Taking health advice from social media is like taking it from a bloke down the pub. Check it out. Chat forums like Health Unlocked allow you to talk to people with similar health questions to your own, but again look out for ill-informed or biased advice.

It boils down to this: the internet is great for background but not for diagnosis. You need a doctor to do that.

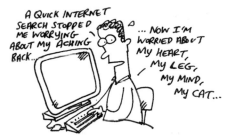

A QUICK INTERNET SEARCH STOPPED ME WORRYING ABOUT MY ACHING BACK... ... NOW I'M WORRIED ABOUT MY HEART, MY LEG, MY MIND, MY CAT...

## Is it OK to buy drugs online?

If you have a prescription from a GP, many GPs and pharmacists can deal with these online.

If you don't have a prescription, get one. Many sites offering drugs without prescription are illegal. The drugs they sell may be useless or dangerous fakes. Plus your credit card details may be stolen.

Perhaps even more importantly, you won't get a diagnosis of your problem. For example, not being able to get an erection won't kill you. But heart disease or diabetes (of which erection problems are a sign) can.

---

## How to avoid colds and flu

Colds and flu are viral infections. Viruses spread easily. If you've got one, you may be infectious from before symptoms appear until they've all gone. Typical symptoms include: runny or blocked nose, sore throat, head ache, muscle ache, cough, sneezing and raised temperature. It's coughing and sneezing that spread viruses. They can live for days on some surfaces, especially in lower temperatures. You can reduce your risk of catching one by:

- washing your hands regularly (soap and water all over);
- avoiding sharing towels etc;
- not touching your eyes and face other than after washing your hands;
- using the hand-gel as you go in and out of GP surgeries or hospitals;
- staying well (in other words, following the tips in this book).

If you've got a virus, avoid passing it onto others. Again it's about hand washing and sneezing into tissues (and binning them as soon as you can). No tissue? Sneeze into your elbow. Don't just sneeze.

Rest, keep warm (viruses don't like it hot), drink plenty of fluids and take over-the-counter treatments from the pharmacist if you need.

Flu tends to come on more quickly and hit you harder than a cold including making you very tired. But the same advice applies. The flu vaccine which is available on the NHS each year to those at particular risk helps prevent flu but not colds.

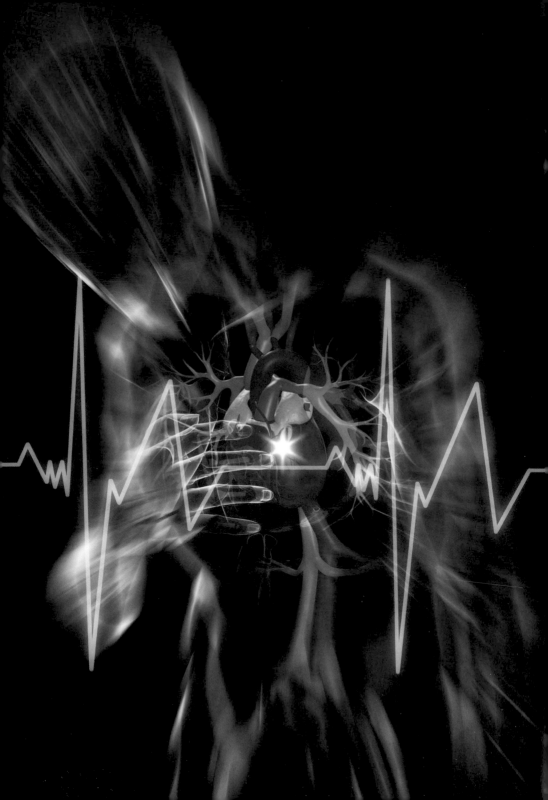

# Am I having a heart attack?

If you take on board the information in this book, you'll definitely reduce your chances of ever having a heart attack. Nevertheless, despite recent improvements, heart disease remains – along with cancer – one of our biggest killers. It makes sense to be prepared.

There are over a million male heart attack survivors in the UK. The British Heart Foundation estimate that the UK survival rate for heart attacks today is about 7 in 10. Not bad odds but – and this is a very big but – a lot of people who survive a heart attack do so because they have it in hospital and all the help is on hand. If you have one outside a hospital, you need to react quickly.

You're far more likely to have a heart attack if you:

■ Have a waist over 94 cm (37 inches)
■ Smoke
■ Take no exercise.

## What are the symptoms of a heart attack?

The most common symptom of a heart attack is central chest pain spreading perhaps to the arms, neck or jaw. You may also feel sick, sweaty or breathless.

Less common symptoms include a 'heavy' feeling or milder discomfort in the chest, more like severe indigestion, that makes you feel generally unwell. You may feel light-headed or dizzy.

If you suspect someone is having a heart attack, you need to get them to hospital as soon as possible. Call 999 immediately and ask for an ambulance. Don't worry about being wrong. Better an honest mistake than paramedics arriving too late. Any paramedic will tell you this.

Outside the UK, 112 is the standard emergency number across the EU and in many other countries. In North America, it's 911. Make sure you know how to call the emergency services from your mobile.

Chewing on a 300mg (adult-size) aspirin might help stop further blood clots.

## Anything else I can do?

Is there a defibrillator nearby? The 999 call handler will be able to tell you.

A defibrillator gives a high-energy electric shock to the heart to jolt it out of cardiac arrest. You've seen the sort of thing on hospital dramas. Public access

### HEART ANATOMY

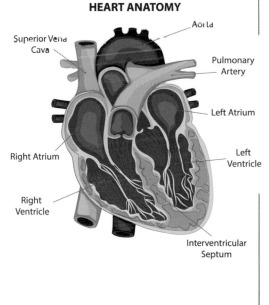

Superior Vena Cava
Aorta
Pulmonary Artery
Left Atrium
Right Atrium
Left Ventricle
Right Ventricle
Interventricular Septum

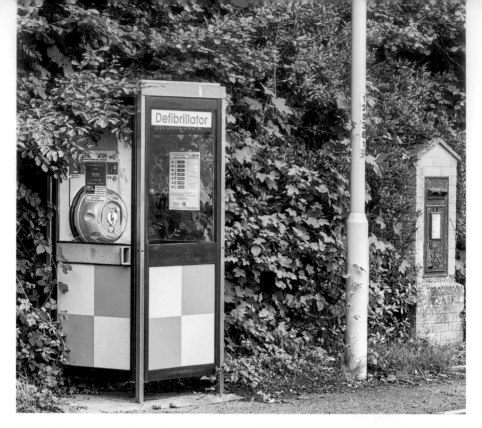

defibrillators can sometimes be found in workplaces and public spaces like airports, train stations, shopping centres and occasionally in the street.

You can also learn how to do cardiopulmonary resuscitation (CPR). This involves pressing up and down on the chest of someone in cardiac arrest to help pump the blood around their body. You can find training videos and more information online.

## How good is the NHS at treating heart attacks?

Mike, the doctor in the box opposite, had his heart attack in New Zealand. But what would have happened to him in the UK on our NHS?

The key measure is the so-called 'call to balloon' (CTB) time: the time between

alerting emergency services (999) and the start of treatment to reopen the blocked

### What are the symptoms of a stroke?

There is an acronym: FAST for remembering the symptoms of a stroke:

**F** = Face is drooping on one side – ask the person to smile.

**A** = Arms are weak or numb – ask the person to raise both of them.

**S** = Speech is difficult to understand or slurred – ask the person to repeat a simple sentence.

**T** = Time to call 999 if you see any of the above.

artery. Research suggests that in 2017–18, 70.5% of NHS patients had a CTB time of under two and a half hours (150 minutes) – the national target – with 44% getting treatment within two hours like Mike.

However, the CTB time is increasing because, it appears, of increased travel times to hospital. This may reflect traffic and availability of ambulances. Once through the hospital door, treatment times are pretty consistent with nearly 9 in 10 patients getting the treatment they need within 90 minutes. In other words, get to the hospital as quickly as possible.

## CASE STUDY

# MIKE: THE GP WHO HAD A HEART ATTACK AT 55

I went to the gym. There were only three guys there, all in their early twenties. I should have thought twice. We did a major workout. The other guys were all sweltering and were amazed I'd kept up. So was I.

As I got in the car, the pain began. By the time I got home, I was holding the steering wheel with one arm and poking my chest. It was quite tender. I thought I'd pulled a muscle, hurt my ribs. Or got indigestion. My wife called the ambulance.

I still wasn't convinced it was a heart attack until I saw the ECG the paramedics did. I had two stents in within two hours. One of my colleagues did it.

I was low on risk factors like blood pressure and cholesterol: waist is just under 36 inches; my BMI was 23.5. Usually up to 25 is considered OK but for Indians some doctors think you should revise it down to 23.

You feel pretty vulnerable as a patient. It was quite sobering. The weekend before, I'd been camping with my family on an island. If it had happened there… well, I figure I've been given a second chance.

I've treated people with heart attacks, but you feel it's never going to happen to you. I've always used stress as a motivator. Indeed, I've enjoyed being calm in stressful situations. But I wonder now if doing this regularly has been bad for me. I'll never know the answer.

*Two years on and with four stents, Mike is living proof that a heart attack, promptly treated, need not be the end of the world:*

Now I do less intense exercise. More social, more all-round activities like swimming and walking. I recently walked 500km in 20 days with a friend. One of the biggest determinants of longevity has nothing to do with hearts or anything. It's about how connected you are with other people.

I have tried to reduce stress in my life. Something like this prompts you to focus on what you want to do in the future as you're aware that your time on the planet is limited.

I think it has made me a better doctor. I am more understanding of my patients and their difficulties.

# Am I addicted?

We live in a world of increasingly scarce resources, yet it doesn't always feel like that. In fact, we seem to be able to get pretty much anything, whenever we want. The problem of too much – even of a good thing – is a problem like never before.

Drinking, illegal drugs, prescription drugs, gambling, slot machines, sex, porn, masturbation, having affairs, your work, your phone, gaming, sport, exercise, smoking, eating, not eating, coffee, sugar, shopping, shoplifting, plastic surgery, tattoos… the list of possible addictions goes on. Some are more serious than others. Some are more likely to kill you than others. The point is, there are many activities that some people do quite happily on and off for their whole lives that others, sooner or later, become addicted to. How do you tell the difference?

- **Preoccupation** – You're thinking about the activity even when you're not doing it. You begin to see people in terms of how they relate to your habit – 'drug buddies'
- **Escalation** – You need more to get the same buzz, or you need to do it for longer and longer
- **Cost** – Your habit is beginning to cost you more than just the cost of the drink, drugs or whatever it is, and is affecting your relationships and family life
- **Absorption** – You lose track of time when you're doing it.

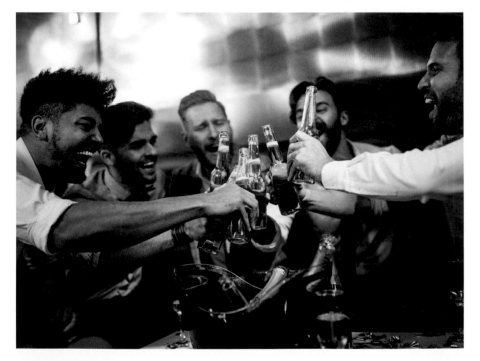

- **You've tried to stop or cut down and you can't** – You're impatient and easily angered when you can't do it for a while
- **You're lying to others about what exactly it is that you're doing** – Playing down your drinking or your gambling losses, for example
- **Escape** – You're aware that you're doing what you're doing to change the way you feel or avoid something

People often try to draw their own lines in the sand to kid themselves that they don't have a problem – 'I'm OK because I don't drink in the mornings.' 'I'm OK because I don't do drugs at work.' 'I'm OK because I only have a bet at the weekends.'

Then the lines start to move. One day it becomes: 'I'm OK because I don't do it on a Sunday in a leap year when the moon's in Uranus and West Ham are at home,' but deep inside you know you have a problem.

If you can, talking to family and friends might help, but this is not always easy. Talking to a professional might be easier. GPs are used to pointing people in the right direction for help with their addiction.

Or there are support groups for people in the same boat. Alcoholics Anonymous, with its 12-step path to recovery, is one option, and has helped many people. There are other groups with similar or different approaches for other addictions including gambling, sex and drugs.

There is no shame in being an addict, even to something that might disgust or appal you. It could happen to anyone. Seek help. The favourite gag of the recovering addict is that denial is not just a long river in Africa. Denial is the barrier between you and recovering your freedom.

## Is vaping better than smoking?

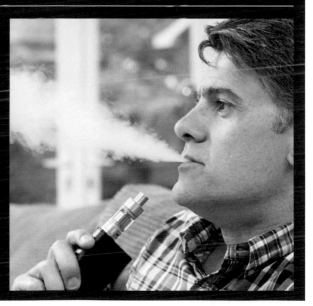

E-cigarettes are not all hot air – they are a regulated product. If you smoke, vaping may be a step in the right direction. But you're still feeding a nicotine addiction, meaning it's easier to slip back into the tobacco habit.

Research continues on the effects of vaping. Clearly, it's highly unlikely to turn out to be as dangerous as smoking but it's also unlikely to have no risk whatsoever.

The NHS offers practical support to quit smoking.

# Warning lights: physical health

The best judge of how you're feeling is you, provided you're being honest with yourself. That's sometimes harder than it sounds. We may put others' health before our own or not want to waste time (ours or the doctor's). We may mistake our hope that something will clear up on its own for certainty that it will. Don't risk it.

Go to the GP if you:

- Lose weight and don't know why
- Lose your appetite
- Have a sore or ulcer that does not heal
- Have a nagging cough or hoarse breathlessness that won't go away
- Cough or vomit blood
- Can't pee comfortably (e.g. if you are in pain, can't start or can't stop, want to pee a lot, or don't feel properly empty afterwards)
- Have unusual discharges from any orifice (especially the penis or backside)
- Have unusual growths or lumps on any part of the body
- Have a mole on the skin that is changing shape (or colour), growing, bleeding or weeping
- Have frequent changes in bowel habit – bouts of constipation or diarrhoea
- Have signs of blood (red or dark black) in your faeces
- Have regular erection problems
- Have pain in any part of the body that won't go away or keeps coming back – this is especially important if the pain is in your chest.

None of these symptoms are particularly pleasant anyway, so it makes sense to get them sorted. They could all also be signs of something more serious that you need to get checked out. Just do it.

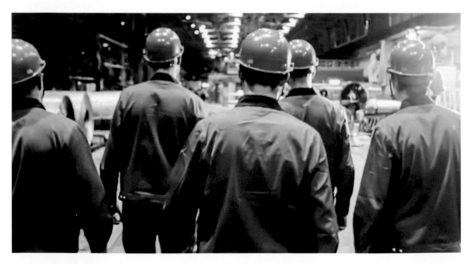

# Warning lights: mental well-being

There's a lot about boosting our well-being at the start of this book. These symptoms are some of the signs that pressure might be building. Treat them like warning lights on the dashboard. Keep an eye out for them.

- Eating more or less than normal
- Mood swings
- Low self-esteem
- Feeling tense or anxious
- Not sleeping properly (or wanting to sleep all the time)
- Poor memory or forgetfulness
- Excessive drinking and/or drug use
- Feeling really tired and lacking in energy
- Withdrawing from family and friends
- Behaving out of character

- Finding it hard to concentrate and struggling at work
- Losing interest in things you usually enjoy
- Having unusual experiences, like seeing or hearing things that others don't or which you know cannot be real
- There may be physical signs too, like headaches, irritable bowel syndrome or aches and pains.

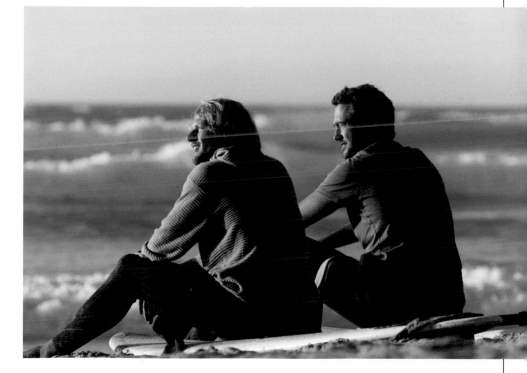

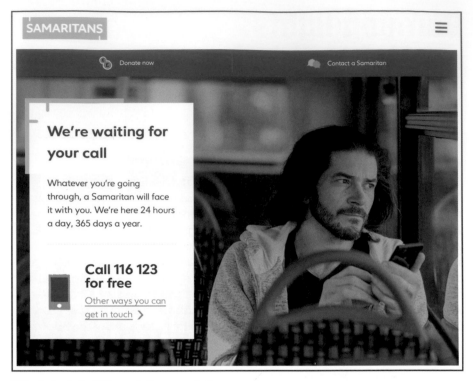

**SAMARITANS** ≡

Donate now    Contact a Samaritan

## We're waiting for your call

Whatever you're going through, a Samaritan will face it with you. We're here 24 hours a day, 365 days a year.

### Call 116 123 for free

Other ways you can get in touch >

## What do I do if I spot the mental wellbeing warning lights?

If you've tried the things that you know generally make you feel better and perhaps a few of the other things in this book and the lights are still flashing, talk to someone. It could be family or friends, if you have someone you can be really honest with.

If you think you need to talk to a professional, your GP can help. Or you might be able to go to a local mental health service without going through your GP.

Sometimes it's easier to talk to someone who doesn't know you. Samaritans are not just for people who feel suicidal. You can talk to their volunteers anonymously about anything that's on your mind at any time at all by phone, email or text. You can even walk in to a branch and talk face to face. Samaritans can also signpost you to other organisations.

Helplines or local support groups also enable you to talk with people who understand a bit about what's on your mind but don't know you personally.

If you'd rather not talk, write: letters or emails you never send; a long rant; a journal or diary; stories or poems; notes; single words. Just writing it down gets it out of you. That feels better. But through writing you're also adding a structure. This might help you understand what you're feeling too.

If you want something to trigger your thoughts, you can buy journals that ask questions and leave blank spaces for you to answer them. What words describe your feelings? What do you think is making you feel like this? How would you like things to be?

# Screen tests

When it comes to health, prevention is best. If you can't prevent a problem, then finding it as soon as possible is second best. That's what screening is for.

Health screening is the future. It's not just for women. Men are entitled to several screening tests too. It varies with age. Ask your GP for more information.

### Age 40: NHS Health Check

The NHS offers men (and women) aged 40–74 a free NHS Health Check every five years, designed to spot early signs of stroke, kidney disease, heart disease, diabetes or dementia. People are invited by letter but if one doesn't arrive, contact your GP directly and ask for a Health Check. If you haven't got a GP at 40, it's time to get one.

### Age 55: Bowel Scope Test

The NHS are rolling out a one-off test at age 55 to inspect your bowel for warning signs of cancer.

### Age 60: Bowel Cancer Home Screening

Men (and women) aged 60–74 are automatically sent an NHS bowel home testing kit every two years. People over 75 can request one.

### Age 60: Free Eye Tests

Anyone aged 60 and over can have a free NHS eyesight test from an optometrist as often as they need one – for most people, this is every two years. This is important because there are several potentially serious conditions that are more common in older people, such as cataracts, glaucoma and macular degeneration. All

are much easier to treat if detected sooner rather than later. Older people are also more likely to need glasses for reading.

### Age 65: AAA Screening

AAA (abdominal aortic aneurysm) is a heart problem. Men (and only men) aged 65 are offered NHS screening for AAA. A quick, painless ultrasound scan of the tummy checks for a bulge or swelling in the aorta, the main blood vessel from the heart. This can be serious if it's not spotted early: it could get bigger and eventually burst. Most men need only one test. Men over 65 who have not been screened before can also ask for a test.

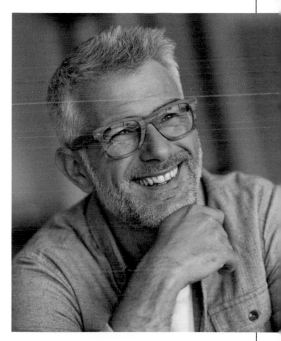

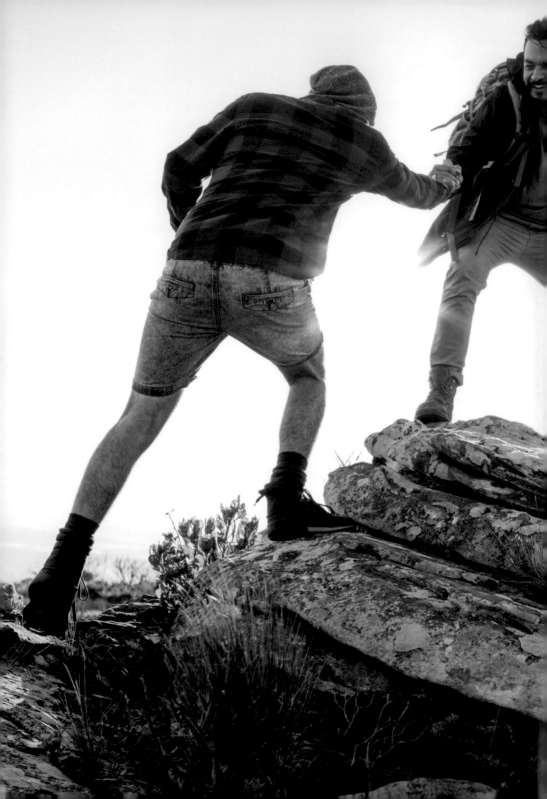

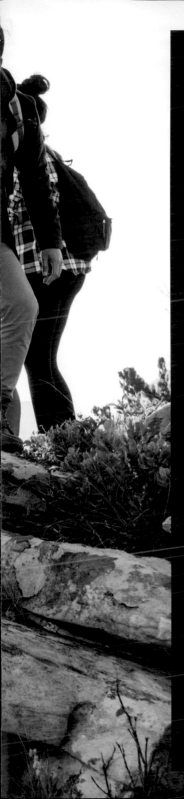

# Last word

When I talk to people about men's health I often mention two mates of mine. I've mentioned them in this book already.

First, there's Phil. Shortly before he died I interviewed him about his bowel cancer. The treatment was tough and he knew the outcome was uncertain.

'All of this might have been avoided had I gone to the GP sooner,' he said. 'I delayed it because I thought I knew what the problem was. I'd had a bad back for a while, which everyone had told me was probably a slipped disc. I was still playing rugby, hooker, and I didn't want to stop playing. I knew I'd miss my rugby. And I was right.'

In his head, he'd downplayed the symptoms that didn't fit in, like needing to go to the toilet all the time. Now I don't know if Phil going to see his GP sooner would have made a difference. Nobody does. But I know I speak for everyone who knew him when I say that I wish he had.

Second, there's Mike. He had a heart attack after overdoing the exercise. The full story is on page 129. Because he's a doctor, he should have known what to do. But because he's a bloke he couldn't believe it was happening to him. He was the man who provided help, not the man who needed it. The bloke in him trumped the doctor and it was down to his wife to call the ambulance.

Enough said?

The message I'll leave you with is this: don't think ill health won't happen to you and don't be a bloke about it if it does. Meanwhile, make a few small little changes that will help make it less likely.

# Useful contacts

If you're looking for health information, the best places to start are the NHS website and the Men's Health Forum website. Both sites include plenty of links to other useful sources of info. I'm also listing some other organisations here (it doesn't mean Haynes or I recommend them; we haven't used them all).

If you want to talk to people with similar health issues to your own, Health Unlocked (healthunlocked.com) is a social network of health communities, including illness and symptom-specific groups. The Forum runs communities on 'men's health' generally and 'penis health' specifically.

If you have a medical problem and aren't sure what to do, contact NHS 111. Call 111 or go online at 111.nhs.uk You can also download the NHS App for your smartphone.

## Alcohol

Drinkaware: www.drinkaware.co.uk
Alcoholic Anonymous:
    www.alcoholics-anonymous.co.uk
Al-Anon (for those affected by
    someone else's drinking):
    www.al-anonuk.org.uk

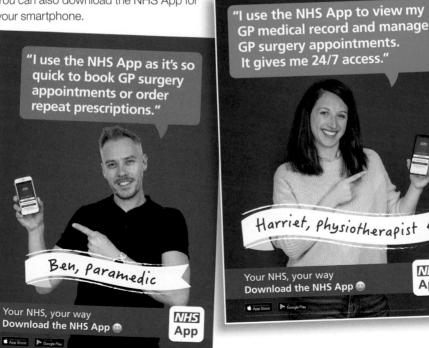

"I use the NHS App as it's so quick to book GP surgery appointments or order repeat prescriptions."

Ben, paramedic

Your NHS, your way
Download the NHS App 😊
App Store   Google Play
NHS App

"I use the NHS App to view my GP medical record and manage GP surgery appointments. It gives me 24/7 access."

Harriet, physiotherapist

Your NHS, your way
Download the NHS App 😊
App Store   Google Play
NHS App

## Cancer

Beating Bowel Cancer:
    www.bowelcanceruk.org.uk
Cancer Research UK:
    www.cancerresearchuk.org
Macmillan Cancer Support (for anyone
    with a cancer diagnosis):
    www.macmillan.org.uk
Orchid (penile, testicular and prostate
    cancer): orchid-cancer.org.uk
Prostate Cancer UK:
    prostatecanceruk.org

## Carers

At least 40% of the UK's unpaid carers
are men.
Carers UK: carersuk.org

## Dementia

Alzheimer's Society:
    alzheimers.org.uk
Dementia UK: dementiauk.org

## Diabetes

Diabetes UK: www.diabetes.org.uk

## Disability

Disability Rights UK:
    www.disabilityrightsuk.org

## Drugs

Frank: www.talktofrank.com
Adfam (families, drugs and alcohol):
    adfam.org.uk
Narcotics Anonymous: ukna.org

## Domestic violence

Men's Advice Line
    (for men on the receiving end):
    www.mensadviceline.org.uk
Respect (for perpetrators):
    www.respectphoneline.org.uk

## Talking to someone

SAMARITANS are for anyone who needs someone to talk to. It's anonymous and confidential. They listen; they don't judge. They're not just for people thinking of ending their life. Samaritans are there 24 hours a day, 365 days of the year. Call 116 123, email jo@ samaritans.org, write a letter or visit your local branch www.samaritans.org

CALM is a suicide-prevention organisation targeted primarily at men. It offers a helpline (0800 585858 or 0808 8025858 in London) and webchat, 5pm-midnight 365 days a year. www.thecalmzone.net

RELATE, the UK's largest supplier of relationship support, operates from over 350 locations in England and Wales. Each local Relate sets its own charges. www.relate.org.uk

Samaritans are not professional counsellors, they are all volunteers but they are exceptionally well-trained. I don't doubt the volunteers from the other organisations I've listed are well-trained too. (I wouldn't have listed them otherwise.) But I have been unable to verify the training for myself.
There are many other organisations supporting people dealing with particular mental health conditions, addictions or abuse. Search for 'Mental health helplines' on nhs.uk.

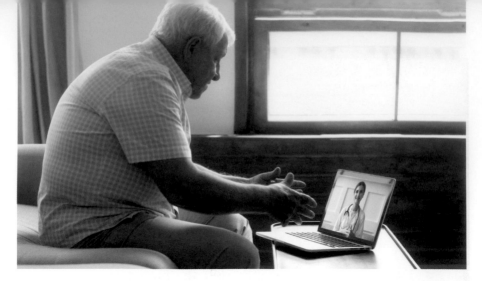

## Eating
Beat (eating disorders):
　　www.beateatingdisorders.org.uk
Man V Fat (weight-loss for men):
　　manvfat.com

## Gambling
GamCare: www.gamcare.org.uk
Gamblers Anonymous:
　　www.gamblersanonymous.org.uk

## Heart and circulation
British Heart Foundation: www.bhf.org.uk
Stroke Association: www.stroke.org.uk

## Mental Wellbeing
Check out the helplines in the box. These
organisations also offer support:
Mind: www.mind.org.uk
Mental Health Foundation:
　　www.mentalhealth.org.uk
Time To Change:
　　www.time-to-change.org.uk

## Organ Donation
*Organ donation saves lives.*
By the end of 2020, England, Scotland
and Wales will all have opt-out systems.
This broadly means that you'll be
considered to have consented to organ
donation unless you opt-out (although
next-of-kin are still involved). Find out more
at: www.organdonation.nhs.uk

## Sexual Consent
Sex without consent freely given is rape:
　　pauseplaystop.org.uk
Stop it Now is for people seeking help with
　　their own abusive behaviour or feelings
　　and those who suspect someone they
　　know presents a risk to children:
　　www.stopitnow.org.uk

## Sexual Health
Terrence Higgins Trust (HIV and sexual
　　health): tht.org.uk
Sex Addicts Anonymous in the UK:
　　saauk.info
There is more information on sexual health
　　on both the NHS and Men's Health
　　Forum sites including links to free
　　condoms.

## Smoking
The NHS has a variety of resources
　　to help with quitting smoking:
　　www.nhs.uk/smokefree
Action on Smoking and Health: ash.org.uk

# The Men's Health Forum

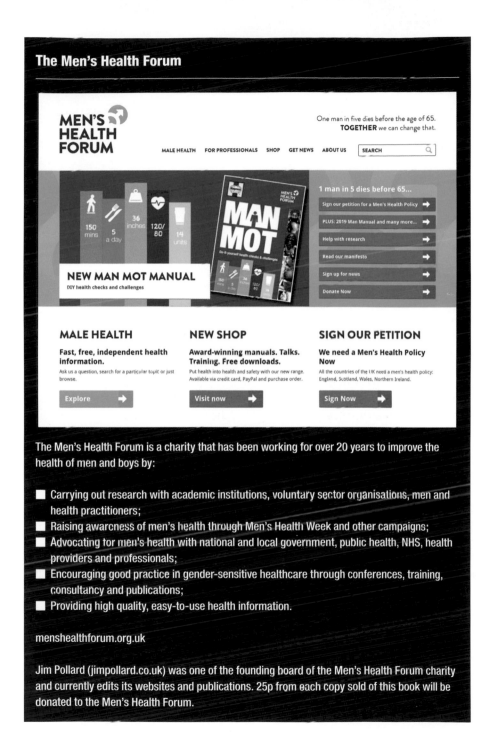

The Men's Health Forum is a charity that has been working for over 20 years to improve the health of men and boys by:

- Carrying out research with academic institutions, voluntary sector organisations, men and health practitioners;
- Raising awareness of men's health through Men's Health Week and other campaigns;
- Advocating for men's health with national and local government, public health, NHS, health providers and professionals;
- Encouraging good practice in gender-sensitive healthcare through conferences, training, consultancy and publications;
- Providing high quality, easy-to-use health information.

menshealthforum.org.uk

Jim Pollard (jimpollard.co.uk) was one of the founding board of the Men's Health Forum charity and currently edits its websites and publications. 25p from each copy sold of this book will be donated to the Men's Health Forum.

# Acknowledgements

Big thanks as ever to all staff and trustees past and present at the Men's Health Forum. Without you men's health wouldn't even be a thing.

A particular nod to the charity's first CEO Peter Baker for letting me cling on to the coattails of his pioneering career for so long and to its first president Dr Ian Banks, the hugely-talented founder of the Forum and effective inventor of men's health journalism.

Thanks to every man who has ever talked to me about his physical or mental health - all umpteen of you - and particularly to those named in this book: Mark, Ian, 'Mike', Steve, Graham and George. Thanks to Sandra for letting me share Phil's words.

Thanks to psychotherapist Tony Williams and ex-copper John Sutherland for talking to me about talking.

Thanks to all the health professionals who have had to put up with me down the years for their exemplary professionalism in the face of the dual provocations of my daft questions and the shocking underfunding of the NHS. I'm sure all parties wish we hadn't had to see quite so much of each other as we have.

Thanks to the team at Haynes for making this book possible and for the support they and indeed the entire Haynes family right up to the very top have given to men's health over the years.

Thanks to Bela for everything (and particularly, in the context of this book, the bits on France and food.)

Thanks to Johan Cryuff for total football.

# Index